ACKNOWLEDGEMENTS

To my wife, Nancy, without your strength, wonderful outlook on life, and your fighting attitude, this book would have never been published.

And to the bravest women I have ever met from Healing Odyssey 13, a cancer recover support group in Laguna Hills, California. Your positive praise and encouragement kept me going so this book could move forward.

I0022312

TABLE OF CONTENTS

Healing From Within

EMOTIONALLY SURVIVING CANCER

BOOK #2

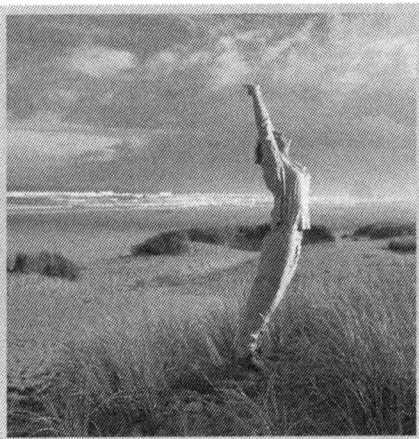

mind diet

Steve Jaffe

THE
MIND
DIET®
GROUP, INC.

Healing From Within, Emotionally Surviving Cancer.

Copyright© 2002 by The Mind Diet Group, Inc.

Printed and bound in the United States of America. All rights reserved.
No part of this book may be reproduced in any form or by any electronic
or mechanical means including information storage and retrieval systems
without permission in writing from the publisher, except by a reviewer,
who may quote brief passages in a review.

ISBN: 0-9720605-1-0

Mind Diet®, is a registered trademark of MDG, the Mind Diet Group, Inc.
and should not be used or reproduced without written permission from
the owner. When referred to in an article or review, the trademark symbol
must appear.

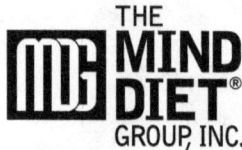

Published by

THE
MIND
DIET®
GROUP, INC.

2217 Levante Street
Carlsbad, CA 92009

Tel: 760.436.7253
Fax: 760.436.6608

E-mail: Aminddiet@aol.com
Web: www.aminddiet.com
www.aminddiet.com

Part Three
THE WORK BEGINS

Part Four
THE EMOTIONAL CURE

A NOTE BEFORE YOU
TAKE YOUR JOURNEY

This book was designed to assist you in finding an easier alternative in dealing with life as it is for you today. Healing from within is extremely appropriate for what you will accomplish as you let go of your fears, anxieties and, most of all, the thoughts of death that stay bottled-up inside your mind. I can't promise you a cure for your illness, however I can promise you that you can learn to live each day happier, and with more understanding toward the life long curse that has been cast upon you.

Each of us copes with our internal and external tribulations differently, uniquely. However, one common thread remains consistent through all of us as our thoughts, stresses, and bodies accumulate excessive pounds of worry, guilt, anxiety, fear, sadness, loneliness, pain, and other negative energies. Unless these issues are dealt with, health problems can surface.

After experiencing some of the most stressful situations in my life, I've come to understand and believe that stress can kill. If not kill, then bring to the surface diseases that may permanently harm your health.

Life was not meant to be easy, nor should it be. How boring things would be for all of us if we did not have emotions or situations that challenged us. Having a life threatening disease like cancer, will continue to challenge you the rest of your life. We have inside our bodies, good emotions and bad emotions. There is good stress and there is bad stress. Unfortunately, our minds and bodies don't always distinguish which stress factors are good for us and which ones are harmful to us. Our problems lie within our present life styles, such as occupation, family structure, relationships and other tasks we place in the large "bucket" we label "worry" and carry it around with us every day. We tend to ignore the unpleasant emotions like weeds just sprouting in a beautiful garden until we eventually allow them to choke the life out of something that was meant to be exquisite.

Throughout this book I will provide guidelines and new gateways for you to enter using rhythm poetry to help you find a positive release. These experiences and newly unconstrained emotions will make your own life's interesting and challenging journey more meaningful. Your present, everyday life should change. I've seen it happen to other cancer survivors. It may not be totally or drastically changed, but it should improve those areas that block you from doing what you truly, deep down inside your soul, want to do, just for YOU. I want this book to open for you new possibilities, potentials and opportunities that weren't there before you opened these pages. At first change will be hard , as this book and its format will be new to you.

Several years ago, during my own personal dark time, my life style was not healthy for me and I felt alone and isolated. It was at that point that I turned to writing poetry. The moment the poems flowed into my heart was the day I began to heal. It was a magical feeling when the honest truth of what I was feeling came to the surface and I put it to a piece of paper. I felt the process blanket my body and help mend my life, which had become too overwhelming.

Sometimes revelations don't come knocking at your door until it's too late. I remember many instances growing up when I stubbornly ignored advice from my parents or teachers. As an adult, I can now see the wisdom in their mentoring. Hindsight is always 20/20 vision; nevertheless, the wisdom and guidance that was lost on me then could have saved a lot of time and grief during an impetuous maturing.

I want to challenge each of you to accept the idea that the Mind Diet form of poetry will work for you. I remember hearing a phrase:

"Poetry is a non-musical form of expression that releases a deep inner part of the soul that needs exercise and excitement."

The Mind Diet form of poetry cannot harm you. What it can do is break down and dissolve the protective masks we all tend to wear throughout our lives, and provide us with an opportunity to re-write our scripts. Wouldn't it be wonderful to have a more peaceful and tranquil day-to-day existence, as you go each day through your recovery process?

I was fortunate to have come to this point in my life during the 1990's when it seemed that everywhere I turned I was locked in frustration and powerless situations. For me it was a decade of challenges that ranged from an ugly divorce, to caring for an ill child, to a major lawsuit with the company I represented as an insurance agent, and finally to losing a career I loved because of my changed health. My body deteriorated from the wear and tear of the stress, which manifested itself in the form of Heart Disease. I spent 1999, in and out of hospitals trying to save my heart from exploding. Finally, on December 3, 1999, I had to have quadruple-bypass surgery. Even though the doctor's prognosis was positive, my mind remained focused on death. No matter how much I tried, a day did not pass that I did not worry about having a fatal heart attack. I thank God I now have my Mind Diet Program, which is my weapon to help me conquer the emotional challenges that lie ahead.

In 1996, I started to write poetry. Not the type of prose a great poet would create. The Mind Diet poems are more like an affirmation form of prose. Some of the poems sound like Mantras, others just sound like pep talks, and some just don't make sense. It really didn't matter at the time I wrote them, as they were just an expression of my emotional state at that point in time. What mattered was that my emotions, those frazzled, locked-up feelings that were killing my body, were being removed and put on paper in a new form of expression. As I became more honest with myself, I opened up the floodgates of pain. Eventually the anguish was put to ink in the form of healing and inspiring words. This new language forced me to deal with my problems and find workable solutions. I found myself writing every day. Usually it was right after I woke up and had my first cup of coffee. What I wrote about carried me forth into my day, helping me over the normal hurdles and challenges that had seemed insurmountable just the day before.

I have to admit, at first poetry didn't help. I was so entrapped within my 'serious' problems, that I believed that they were extremely catastrophic to me and me alone. After dutifully writing my poems without missing a day, it finally happened: a release of pressure. Like air escaping from a balloon, I was able to cope. Well, I cannot tell you how wonderful that experience felt. The tightness in my neck disappeared. My body became relaxed for the first time in many years. My miles of stressful situations began falling like dominos.

It did not take a rocket scientist to tell me that what I was doing was healthy. As I progressed, so did the next step in the evolution of my poems. The phrase "A Mind Diet Experience" had been created to express that magical feeling.

From that day forward I've continued writing my poetry and believe it has helped slow down my heart disease. I will not make any claims that I have reversed it. However, I feel with my new life style changes and my Mind Diet Poetry, I can conquer all the problems that await me down my highway of life.

For me, my life is now a Mind Diet. I live each day as if it were my last and deal with my day-to-day problems with a big smile. I see things that I never could see before. Death doesn't frighten me as it once did. I do not look back and torture myself with what might have been, or "why me" scenarios. When I die, which I know for sure will happen someday – I am ready. I want to look back on my days and have no regrets. I do not want to be sitting in a rocking chair complaining about all the things that I wished I could have done, or the places that I wished I could have seen, or the people I should have known better. Whether I need a walker or a wheelchair to remain active in my world, I will do so with my Mind Diet poems and my new life spirit.

Ask yourself the following questions: "Have I truly seen a sunrise and a sunset on the same day?" "Have I stopped to smell the roses?" Have you really stopped? Most of us in our busy day-to-day schedules see the roses, but never really slow down and smell them. "Have I really tried to know and understand my spouse, significant other, friends, family or children?"

During your journey inside this book you will be invited to experience feelings that you may have had locked away most of your life. Your first inclination will be to skim the surface of what this book can offer you. Then you'll resist the changes that you will need to take to experience a true Mind Diet mindset. Change is very difficult, especially when it's honestly directed at you.

Do not procrastinate, because we all have a designated number of tomorrows to put to good use. Having a life threatening disease, or losing someone close to you, or just not enjoying who you are, can be dealt with through my Mind Diet Program. The first Mind Diet Series Book: *Count Your Life With Smiles Not Tears* focuses on the overall YOU. This book focuses only on cancer. I highly recommend that after completing *Healing From With, Emotionally Surviving Cancer,* that you try my first Mind Diet Series Book. You can find it at my website: aminddiet.com

I recommend that you share your work with people in your life, those who you can trust. By doing so you will be able to witness doors opening up in your relationships that were previously locked.

Inside this book you will find blank *Personal Emotions* pages that will allow you to record the emotional truth that will rise to the surface after each read poem. Either use our Mind Diet Journal or one of your own to record the other Mind Diet experience that you have each day, week, month and year. In fact, you will find that you have been having Mind Diet experiences most of your life, but never noticed them. Inside the journal, you will create through a rhythm form of poetry, a new side of you that will allow you to deal with current and past emotional difficulties. Don't get scared if you can't write poetry; I don't believe I can either. Just write down your feelings and your own personal rhythm will surface. You will begin to find solutions to relationship problems, physical disabilities, and problems in your life that you could not deal with before. Your disease will no longer be the primary issue you think about, thus allowing you to enjoy the life that is waiting for you to re-enter.

Healing From Within, Emotionally Surviving Cancer, interrelates with my other books. It is a guide to removing the excess emotional weight that we all carry around with us, hindering our ability to accomplish the things in our lives that are important. Have you ever wondered why a relationship you were in failed? Why bad things happened to you? Why things just wouldn't go right in your life? *The Mind Diet Series* can help you find a solution that will bring you increased happiness and joy.

This book, combined with your courage, will unleash a hidden part of you that will help you through future difficulties in your life. I encourage you to enjoy the Mind Diet experiences that await you.

THE STRUGGLE FOR ANSWERS AND REASON

If there is a hard part to a problem, then I believe it is our mind's struggle for answers and reasons for the "Unfair Deal" which has been cast upon us. The hearing of shocking news is never rationally or appropriately timed. One morning you may wake up to the day that will turn your life upside down. Your emotions will be put into a type of shock mode and you will instantly try to draw on some past experience, which will allow you to say the right words, act with the correct expressions, and even express your own deeply routed emotions, fittingly. Unfortunately, there are no rulebooks to deal with bad news. It is said, however, that "fear is the beginning of wisdom."

Hearing for the first time that you, or some one close to you has cancer can make you feel as if an elephant has just stepped on your chest.

I myself, experienced that horrible shock on May 12, 1998. That was the day my wife, Nancy, had her biopsy. Her doctor, an emotionless "droid," then told me without expression: *"SHE'S GOT BREAST CANCER. I'll know for sure the results of her biopsy tomorrow, but I've done enough of these procedures to be sure I'm right."* I didn't know what to say to the doctor about her own good news? Her arrogant bragging about being so smart. I almost felt like giving her a high-five slap and congratulating her that she again was right. But, she was talking about my wife, my best friend, the person whom I planned to spend the rest of my life with and if you know me, that's supposed to be longer than eternity. Then she got up and left without a "good-bye" or a "hang-in there, everything will be all right." I just sat there numb, lost with a tornado of thoughts that swirled inside my head. I began to cry, not for my pain, but for what my wife was going to have to go through. What decisions she would have to make and how I was going to be strong for her.

I feel that many doctors must go to "Insensitivity Training 101" as a requirement to be a physician. After feeling the life drain out of me with this horrible news, I tried to get my composure back and ask some important questions, but my tongue seemed tied in knots and I must have sounded like a blithering idiot. I was surprised by the fact that the doctor had left her compassion at home. I just assumed that a female doctor would have been more sensitive to a disease that affects mostly women. I might have understood if a male doctor was being insensitive, but not this one.

Before my mind and my thoughts could straighten out, the doctor had walked away and I was left with the horrible image of my wife dying of breast cancer. The doctor did advise me that Nancy might not remember that she was told this same news right after her surgery. She had been given a drug that was designed to block her memory of the surgery, as well as the doctor's torturous words. I had wished at that time the doctor would have offered me that same pill, so I could forget about our conversation and pretend it never happened. Right at that moment I wished I had been an ostrich.

So there I was, taking Nancy home eight hours later and realizing that besides her doctor, I was the only other person in the world who knew she had breast cancer. My beautiful wife still had that glint of hope in her eyes, that maybe at her appointment the next day, the results of her biopsy would be negative.

I know this may sound superficial, but that was the worst day of my life. I'm not very good at keeping things from her, but after a few large glasses of wine, I had convinced myself that maybe Nancy's optimism was going to work, and the doctor would be incorrect for the first time, and there was not going to be any sign of breast cancer on the pathologist's report.

The next day, I – this macho man, a black belt in Karate – passed out in the examination room when I heard the doctor again say those four horrible words: "You have Breast Cancer." After the nurse and doctor attended to me with looks of disgust, as if I was trying to turn the attention away from my helpless wife, I got back my composure and listened to the diagnosis that has forever changed our lives.

Seeing my Nancy keeping her chin held high, holding back her tears, and acting strong made me think about my poems and how they helped me through my own problems. Oh how I wished right there I could have read a poem and made the tension in the examination room disappear.

I listened to the doctor, listened to Nancy's questions and then listened to her fears and anger on our thirty-minute drive home from the doctor's office. I wrote down words, expressions, and personal feelings about my new life change, which had taken place less than twenty-four hours earlier. I asked

Nancy to write her emotions down on a sheet of paper, and anything that was twisting inside her mind about what she was thinking. I'm grateful she didn't rip my head off with all the questions I had asked. While being her nurse, cook and bottle washer, I found time during her naps to create this compilation of Poems.

It had turned out – not by choice or methodology – that I wrote these poems as if it was me who had the cancer. I have enclosed a message that Nancy wanted to include in this book to share with all the women who have survived or are currently struggling with breast cancer, and to their spouses, families, and friends who struggle with them. Nancy is presently very active with many Cancer Support Groups and wants to share something that had helped her.

A LOVING MESSAGE FROM NANCY JAFFE - A CANCER SURVIVOR

"You have CANCER." Those words, spoken to me by my doctor, changed everything in my life forever. Nothing was ever the same after that. Surprisingly, however, life became better than before in many ways, more abundant and precious. However, that didn't happen right away. The emotions that I felt ranged from confusion, fear, anger, curiosity, pain, defeat, and weakness; to comfort, strength, greater spirituality, deeper love and appreciation. As Dolly Parton once said: "If you want the rainbow, you gotta put up with the rain." As I was experiencing all the emotions during diagnosis, surgery, radiation treatments, physical therapy, and recovery; my husband Steve was "feeling" what I was feeling. He began writing these thoughts and feelings down in poetry. Each day he would read me a poem. It helped me to feel as if he really understood what I was going through, and it gave me immense support. Eventually he wrote over 90 poems, and put them all down in this book, entitled *Healing From Within, Emotionally Surviving Cancer*.

I hope this helps you as much as it did me.

– *Nancy Jaffe*

Part One
WHAT IS A MIND DIET EXPERIENCE?

You are probably wondering, "what does a Mind Diet have to do with breast cancer?" It has everything to do with it. If you're reading this book you may be recovering from your shock of the initial diagnosis, the pain from radiation and chemotherapy treatments, and/or possibly the physical therapy, which Nancy told me was pure torture. You may now be taking medications that affect your body, medications that are causing your body to become a stranger to you.

From uncontrolled hot flashes, to fatigue, again back to uncontrolled hot flashes, oh... again back to fatigue... you now find yourself looking at your life and wondering for the first time if you have enough seconds, minutes, hours, days, months, or years to do what you hoped to do before retirement. With the *Mind Diet Program,* you "retire" today. Not really retire, specifically in the traditional sense. *The Mind Diet Experience* will open up opportunities that you never knew existed, and you'll be kept busier than you've ever been. Your life has changed forever, so why not begin with a new attitude?

Can you remember a time in your life when warm fuzzy feelings were blanketing your body regularly? Think very hard, because that feeling is what I mean by a Mind Diet. Do you remember the last time you laughed? Not just a giggle or a chuckle, but a real hard belly laugh that brought tears that messed up your make-up and made your nose drip like a leaky faucet? That's a Mind Diet.

Do you remember your first kiss? Or the first time you completed a hard project and received accolades from the one person whom you wanted to please? That's a Mind Diet.

Anything that allows you to feel euphoric, goose-bumpy, warm-cuddly, or plain, old, down to earth happy, that's a Mind Diet.

I'm sure your doctors have told you to think about life style changes to enhance your chances for a full recovery. What the Mind Diet Series Books helps you do is enhance the needed changes in your life, eliminate the negative stresses, and help you along to a successful remission. Think of this book

1

as a treatment manual that will work in tandem with all your other recovery treatments.

This book will help you deal openly and honestly with the negative stresses in your life and put you in a better place to fight the meanest word in the English language: cancer.

As you read these poems, jot down your feelings. Ask yourself: How do I relate to the words in the poem? Then when you feel strong, write yourself a poem in your Mind Diet Journal. The rhythm and form don't matter. It's the writing and putting your feelings down on the paper that counts. Remember, at first it didn't work for me, either. But when your own rhythm clicks, you will not be able to stop!

When you feel safe and comfortable, read your poem to someone who loves you and will not judge you. Then let them read the poem on their own. What you'll experience is a completely new form of communication that will open up many new doors for that relationship. Understand that "outsiders," (people who don't have your disease), don't know what to say or do to help you. The Mind Diet Experience, your poetry, can break down that barrier and bring them closer to you than they have ever been before.

There is only one rule you need to remember when reading and writing your Mind Diet Poetry: There are no rules, so enjoy! Have a million Mind Diet Experiences and see what awaits you in your new world.

Below is a brief guideline to help you remain focused and on track when writing your poetry. Remember, THERE ARE NO RULES:

BASIC RULES TO HAVING A TRUE MIND DIET

1. There are no rules to finding your own Mind Diet Rhythm.

2. Be sure to read each of these poems at least twice before writing down your own poem or written emotions.

3. Your poems do not have to sound or be close to the poems in this book. I have my own style and you will find your style.

4. Share each poem with a loved one or friend, and share your poems with them when you feel safe and secure.

5. Try to have your loved one or friend write you a poem or a short description of their feelings after they have read the subject poem and your poem.

6. Always allow time to communicate your feelings about the poems and allow time for your loved one or friend to communicate their feelings about what they heard and wrote.

7. Write poems in many locations. At doctors offices, treatment facilities, parks, the beach, your home, hospital, even work.

8. Force yourself to write a poem during the worst of times and the best of times.

9. Listen for your rhythm and observe how it changes over time. You'll begin to notice that your feeling and emotions might start out with the problem, but will finish with a positive solution.

10. Don't get discouraged at first; it takes time to feel better. You don't lose 20 pounds on a diet immediately, so don't expect your Mind Diet to be immediate. Results should be slow, but noticeable.

11. Write as many poems as you can about how you are feeling at the moment. A good sign is when you go beyond the exercises and just want to write.

12. Don't forget to set your goals to be honest and truthful with yourself, so you and only you can find that wonderful person that has remained locked up inside your head.

There are no limits to how you go about your own Mind Diet. Remember, your view on life will always be different than someone else's. Respect yourself and others at all times

"GO AWAY I AM NOT HOME"

I know there's something happening inside, I can sense a change in me, I hear a knocking at my door, afraid to get up and see. I am not ready to be disturbed, my life is just fine as it is, so go away I am not home, this time is controlled by me.

The knocking continues, it drives me insane, I force myself up to see, a doctor waits outside my door, the fear builds up in me. Go away I am not home, come back another time, I am not ready to talk to you, I feel just great, I'm fine.

The fear continues, I know what's wrong, I just can't face it right now, I need a little more time to reflect, before It breaks my bow. These words have meaning that scare me so, I lack the knowledge of what it all means, I try to allow my thoughts to be in control, this fear just overwhelms me.

It's 'Cancer' I hear, which makes me think: "Death", the tears just fill my soul, maybe there was a mistake that the results were wrong, this is not my time to go. There was no mistake, the results were correct, I have now become part of a group, my life will change as I journey today, with the fear that has come into my room.

I have a choice as part of this group, to be one of the success stories you hear, or just give up and allow this disease, to take control of my thoughts and my fears.

The choice will be made by the person I am, and the support from the people around, but the results will succeed when I choose to move forward and conquer this problem I've found. No matter the course or the actions to take, I'll go forward to win at all costs, my life is too precious to give up and die without a fight, and not showing myself who's the boss.

Personal Emotions

"REARRANGE YOUR CLOSET"

*The news was bad, you feel like you were just hit with a two-by-four,
the tears roll down your cheeks so fast, control seems out the window
for evermore, the confusion is taking over at last.*

*You feel like time is short right now, no time to plan and think,
if it's all over don't worry anymore, let the mess just rot and stink.
But if you care to fight real hard then take the steps to journey on,
and begin to rearrange you life today, the fun has just begun.*

*Your life today has been given, a new outlook for you to see,
that life is precious each day you're here, its wonders are ready to be.
Ask yourself have you done all that you want, or is work still on your mind,
well maybe it's time to rethink your priorities
and choose to have a really good time.*

*Your past routine no more defines you, or can be re-lived as it
once was, it's today with tomorrows that's in your plans,
this will now be your new job.
There still is life that can be enjoyed, with minimal change for you,
just rearrange some old priorities, to help you travel through.*

*Place what was past inside your closet, and put plastic around it tight,
and bring out in the open to see, the things you know are
colorful and bright. Today you move with different eyes, and move with
different goals, but understand that how you move, is so
precious for you to hold. To rearrange your life today, puts what you want
in control, and brings to you a needed purpose, that you can see and hold.*

*It requires thinking deep inside your heart to see a waiting playful circus,
and follow everyday the light, that now becomes your
purpose. Plan as if you have, a need to do, the things that
dreams were once just thoughts, and go into your closet today and take
out those wants before they're all lost.*

*This is just your awakening that life for you, needs to be just what you
want it to be, and all that is happening around you now is the foundation
for tomorrow's jubilees. Take time to reflect on all your past ways it is
what you were back then, and take the dreams you always had, and
make them your new best friend.*

Personal Emotions

"THE BOXER"

Your notice was delivered, a challenge has been made, you have been chosen to fight for your life, the opponent you face is a formidable foe, who can permanently turn off your lights.

The fear in your heart for the loss that awaits, flows through you with lightning speed. Your body becomes like a jell-o mold all wobbly for all to see, you try to run away from your fight to avoid what might just be.

Training is needed, to condition your mind and build strength where your heart needs to go, so gather the facts of the fight that you have, to develop the punches that flow. Each fight that was past, can be won easily, if you look for the weaknesses that are there, and don't let your opponent put fear in your mind or his victory will put you on your rear.

The past tell us ways that your opponent has lost and the ways that your opponent has won, but clearly the victories you need for this fight is the attitude that IT can be won. Your opponent only wins when the fear inside you, does not allow you to challenge each move, and you take all the punches that damage your heart, making you appear all black and blue.

Don't show all your fear, but the anger you have, and stare at your opponent straight on, and offer right back your positive attack with a series of punches that move him beyond. Keep your punches real hard, with the attitude you're tough and the pride in your heart that you will win, and see the fear inside of your opponent's eyes as he begins to lose his fight from within.

Each round that you face will begin to turn for you and the right punch will be ready to land, and wait for the moment when the right opening will appear, with your victory wrapped tight in your hand.

Personal Emotions

"MAKE LOVE TO ME MY WAY"

Inside of me my soul is burning,
with the Cancer that has entered me now.
I'm moving around in a dizzy state,
not seeing my future too well.
I need you more than ever before,
but not like we did yesterday,
so please understand with the touch of my hand
that you need to make love just my way.

As my body gets probed and cut with the knife,
that's helping me fight what's inside,
I need to avoid other probes just right now,
and just lie in our bed by your side.
I need you more than ever before,
but not like it was yesterday,
I need you to see the changes inside
and not feel rejected or turn away.

Please make love to me my way,
with hugs and kisses true,
and never look away as I change.
Just hold my hand and walk with me,
each day and night, and talk.
I want our future so very bright,
as I continue to cry and moan,
I want my love to find a new place,
that in my sick body I now call home.

With all my heart and soul, I will come back to you,
and make love as best I can.
And promise you, that if you make love to me my way,
I can survive, oh yes I can.

Personal Emotions

"MY PRIVATE PLACE"

I've always needed a place for me,
for the thoughts that flowed through my head,
but now it's required even more as I heal, and deal
with the emotions that make me mad.
Don't ever think I'm gone from the place,
we call our home or the life we share everyday.
Just try to understand that this place is special for me
to discover the new person I am.
I need to know you see inside of me,
the need for this place that's my own,
and I will return each day with the thanks,
for letting me be on my own.

Inside my private place,
I deal with thoughts of my life,
it could include what we have together,
or the illness that's captured my life.
So when I enter my place for me
with no time limits or distraction to embrace,
please find some things to occupy your time,
so when I walk on out,
I will see smiles not frowns on your face.

If we can find this place for me,
during a time that has halted our flow,
I'll come back to you with thanks from my heart,
I promise the feelings will show.

Personal Emotions

"WHAT PART OF THE GROUP AM I IN?"

I have been called by name to be part of a group,
that I really don't want any part of,
but I am unclear as to what part I am going to play,
in this group that I have become part of.

So many groups form the club I am in,
with so many different ranks that I can have,
but all of these levels that are available to me
are making me feel very mad.

It's a bad dream that has controlled me now,
and the association just scares me so,
I just want to awake from this horrible nightmare
and go back to the world that I had once known.

So if I must, be part of this nasty group,
let me just be in the group that succeeds,
and take from this group the results that are good,
and go forth with my life that will be.

I will control what part of the group,
I find myself struggling in,
and control the results that I want oh so bad,
to direct the new life that I'm in.

I'll move everyday with a joy in my heart that will
control the cells inside,
and be the one whose in charge of my life,
and show the group I still have my pride.

Personal Emotions

_____
_____
_____
_____
_____
_____
_____
_____
_____
_____
_____
_____
_____
_____
_____
_____
_____
_____
_____
_____
_____
_____
_____
_____

"DAY BY DAY"

Before my days just drifted by,
with plans that seemed so bold,
but now my days are planned for pain,
with emotions that are uncontrolled.
Day by day I drift into, a roller coaster ride,
that keeps me guessing what is next to happen,
and what's my next surprise.

I know to take each day as it comes,
with each result that is given to me,
but deep inside my darkest parts,
my plans seem to be in a state of freeze.
I can't begin to plan tomorrow,
when my thoughts float to my continuing pain,
I want to be in control again,
and see sunshine as my friend.

Day by day I begin to change, from the past
of who I was, forming a person that sees life for me,
much different than it was.
I need to make a list of who,
this new person I want shall be,
and set my goal to reach this image,
day by day so very slowly.

I will set my goals during all this pain
and emotional times I have, and evaluate my progress,
removing the thoughts of things that are so bad.
Day by day I will watch me grow,
into the true person I want for me,
and come through this time of pain and sorrow,
a conqueror for all to see.

Personal Emotions

"EYE OF THE TIGER"

To win at life, with all it's challenges,
you need to want success just for you,
and focus on the things that make you happy
and fight for what is really true.
You need to stare at the challenges you face,
with the eyes that show your power,
and make the challenges turn around and run,
or find a new situation to sour.

The Eye of The Tiger is a focus you need,
a drive that pulls you up, keeping you in continued focus,
so you never try to give up.
Remember your past, when goals you had,
were the goals that succeeded for you,
and see the actions that you had then,
that blindly got you through.

You need a hunger to succeed, a thirst for what is right,
and fight like hell to achieve those goals,
with a mighty forceful fight.
Train real hard, building strength of mind,
with strength of body and soul,
to become The Tiger that awaits for you,
to achieve and gain control.

The Eye of the Tiger is a state of mind, a kind of mental trance,
it allows you to succeed at things you want,
without a second glance.
Remain real focused, doing the best you can,
and never lose sight of your goals,
and the Eye of the Tiger will be there for you,
giving you back your needed control.

Personal Emotions

Personal Emotions

Personal Emotions

Part Two
CREATING A NEW YOU

Now that you have had time to write some poems, discover your hidden emotions, and best of all, experience a Mind Diet, it is time to explore the possibility that you can create a new you.

I'm sure you will agree that your cancer and the medical procedures you have had to endure so far have changed the way you see yourself. I read a long time ago that it is possible to "paint a picture" of yourself through the use of honest, descriptive words or phrases.

In order to bring positive change to your life, you need to honestly evaluate who you are today and who you want to be from this day forward. Cancer has changed your life. This might sound like an understatement, but it's true. However, your disease has opened up a world of possibilities that needs to be explored.

To experience this journey, the first and best thing you can do is to become the real YOU. Your opportunity to start all over is staring you right in the face. The evaluation sheet that I want you to fill-out, will help paint a true picture of the person that is hidden deep inside of you and has not yet come out to enjoy the world. I couldn't think of a better time than now to bring out that person. You've gotten your wake-up call and need to get moving.

The following assignment (Personal Evaluation) will take a big effort on your part and it will be one of your most rewarding.

The way this exercise works is simple: Make a list of the attributes that best describe who you would like to be today. You can use one or two word images to do this. Once you've finished, begin rating each of these attributes on a scale from one to five, with five being the highest positive rating for a characteristic of yourself. Also, when you rate yourself be critical and honest, as this will serve as your baseline.

Each month, re-grade yourself to see if there's been an improvement. If your rating hasn't changed, focus your efforts on a specific area that needs improvement. Use your Mind Diet Journal to write poems describing your weaknesses. Be sure to add a positive affirmation toward the end. It is important to end your poems constructively. Continue to practice working on just one specific weak characteristic each week, with the goal of making a degree of improvement. Once you have achieved your results, move on to the next hurdle and repeat the same process.

After one month, re-grade yourself and compare your rating with the prior one. Keep doing the above steps along with the poems in this book until your total grade is in the nineties. If you can remain at ninety percent or higher, then you've created a new you. Good luck!

PERSONAL EVALUATION FORM (SAMPLE)

Qualities Wanted	Score Date: 1/95	Score Date:	Score Date:
Be Trustworthy	4		
Open About Self	1		
Be More Patient	2		
Be 20lbs Lighter	1		
A New Hair Style	1		
More Outgoing	2		
Less Competitive	3		
Exercise Frequently	1		
Express Feelings Easier	2		
Listen To Other Better	1		
Like Myself Better	1		
Become Stronger Emotionally	2		
Start A Hobby	1		
Find More Personal Time	2		
Become More Charitable	2		
Not Be Afraid To Take Risks	4		
Give All Relationships 110% Of Me	3		
Be Unconditional In My Actions	4		
Explore And Find New Adventures	3		
Have A Smile Everyday	2		
Become More Spiritual	4		
Slow Down And Smell The Roses	2		
TOTAL SCORE	43		

EVALUATING YOUR SCORE

1 = Unfavorable
2 = Below Standards
3 = Average
4 = Above Average
5 = Achieved Quality Desired

ANALYSIS OF TOTAL SCORE

Below 69 = Needs Lots of Work
70 - 79 = Average
80 - 89 = Great Improvement
90 + = You've Made It

PERSONAL EVALUATION FORM

Qualities Wanted	Score Date: _____	Score Date: _____	Score Date: _____
TOTAL SCORE			

EVALUATING YOUR SCORE

1 = Unfavorable
2 = Below Standards
3 = Average
4 = Above Average
5 = Achieved Quality Desired

ANALYSIS OF TOTAL SCORE

Below 69 = Needs Lots of Work
70 - 79 = Average
80 - 89 = Great Improvement
90 + = You've Made It

MAKING THE
NEW YOU WORK

Honesty will release the makeover that has been held back by your desire to remain shut-in your old ways. However, if you've been truthful on your evaluation sheet, that person is now going to disappear. Remember, you are a woman or man with cancer and your life will never be the same again.

I've said it before, but it is worth repeating: Having cancer is not the end of the world. Each day that you're alive is a day that you can make a difference to yourself and the people around you. I have spoken to and been around hundreds of cancer survivors that appreciate how precious their life has become. Don't fall victim to what I call "surface emotions," the false smiles and insincere enthusiasm that can surface. You've painted a new picture of yourself and should shout it out to the world honestly.

The personal evaluation form is a terrific tool to inspire and motivate change. Now may be the first time you have truly understood that you will not live forever. No one can predict the future and that is why we should live in the today's that we all have left.

You've heard the stories before how doctors have given a person with cancer only six months to live and that person has laughed in the faces of all who thought death was on the doorstep and is still living a productive life. That can be you if you are willing to change.

No one should ever give up. Seconds matter. They add up to days, then months and finally to happy years. Redefine yourself today and make it your job to sculpt the person you have always wanted to be, leaving the dread of cancer on the back burner until you are ready to give up, which I hope is never.

The personal evaluation form does work. It has worked for many cancer survivors. It is the key to unlocking that new person of honesty and truth. Continue writing your feelings after reading the all poems on the following pages and look for the beauty in your days and all the Mind Diet experiences you can find.

"MIND DIET ROADWAYS FOR LIFE"

Hello my friends, I see you clear,
the life you offer me,
from pretty flowers all around,
to the sparkling deep blue sea.
You are my soul, the food I need,
to be what my life's about,
I love your rays you shine on me,
it makes me want to shout.

There is no more cement around,
or the stress that work has done,
but just the pleasures of your sights,
to bask in your warm feeling sun.
I came from you many years ago,
and began as I now return,
and apologize for my absence so long,
and ask for another turn.

I will slow down to see your beauty,
bringing it into my heart each day,
and if you allow me many years,
I will appreciate you as I play.
You are my diet, my needed ways,
to see my life be fulfilled,
and I will take in the sights around,
to make me feel quite good.

Personal Emotions

"HOPE IN SMALL BUNCHES"

I know how serious this disease is to me,
but I am also quite serious too,
I want some hope in small doses that say,
my life is not totally through.

I listen for words with the results that I get,
but my doctors won't express the hope for me to see,
they only say the words,
that protect their good name,
not caring about the pain it causes me.

I know no one knows,
what the future will bring,
or the time when this disease will just end,
but I need all the hope that can come to me now,
it has become my new best friend.

So listen to me all the cells that I have,
as you attempt to make me your new home,
I am prepared to fight you very hard,
and suggest you just leave me alone.

I am stronger than you,
with an attitude that will,
be all the hope to destroy who you are,
so move on from my life,
before I choose to fight
and destroy the bad cells that you are.

Personal Emotions

"THOUGHTS OF LOVE"

Alone you're not, so don't feel sad,
we all share the pain you feel,
if only we could divide it up,
so the fear will be less real.
We all love you so,
and know that you,
will come through this truly okay,
and we will be just steps away,
to help you every day.

Our thoughts have power that will combine,
to kill the cells that try to harm,
and break them into little pieces,
that won't be able to cause alarm.
We are a mighty group you see,
that care so much for you,
that tell these evil little cells,
that we won't allow stay with you.

So when you feel so overwhelmed,
with thoughts that give you fits,
just try to remember we are steps away,
to help you out of the pits.
Don't feel that you will burden us,
or cause us to feel pain,
we need to be part of this time with you,
to bring sunshine once again.

Personal Emotions

"GIVING UP IS NOT AN OPTION"

No matter the results or the course of action,
that is needed to win this fight,
giving up will not be a choice,
that you will put in your sights.

A fight for life has many unknowns,
but were there knowns before?
It is your job to do the things,
that keep the life inside your door.
When days seem bleak with pain for you,
it means the fight has results,
and needs your courage to succeed,
to make this all work out.

Giving up is not an option,
nor the way to be prepared,
you need to keep the faith alive,
and never be despaired.
I know the pain you must feel now,
the frustration of your life,
you need to keep your hope around,
to help you stay alive.

Each day that's filled with dark, sad times,
will turn to show you light,
that fighting is the only way,
to make your days be bright.
So giving up is not an option,
that, I will totally agree,
I want you fighting everyday
and be always around with me.

Personal Emotions

"FEEL YOUR LIFE"

Start with a pinch to know you're there,
and look deep inside your eyes,
you have a wonderful life to enjoy,
to fulfill and survive.
No matter the days or the way you feel,
there is a life that will bloom,
it's given to you every hour,
and can be gone from you real soon.

Feel your life, it's changing now,
and can change for you quite well.
The time is now for you to see,
it's not a living hell.
Each day has beauty, just open up,
and look around and see.
The friends you know from before this pain,
are waiting for you to be.

It's attitude, with guts of strength,
that shows you are alive,
and makes you strive for all you're worth,
to keep you satisfied.
So don't give up,
you are still around,
with life that has some worth,
and feel the life each day you have,
it's calling for a new birth.

Personal Emotions

"INSIDE I WAIT FOREVER"

My sentence is set, no matter the results,
I have to wait to know my future.
The mental pain I have to endure,
is something I wish someone else could look after.

I know my luck could be short lived,
or not be luck at all,
but just the waiting every day,
not able to know for sure.
But, before this time I did not know the results,
or the length of future I had,
so what's the difference today has made,
it's similar to the past.

No matter what is wrong with me,
or if my health is fine,
I have to wait inside forever,
to know my own true time.
So if I must be living today,
with what my life deals me,
I will continue to live each day I have,
with love that is for real.

I promise I will wait forever,
to see my candle die,
and hope I live each day fulfilled
with happiness, joy and pride.

Personal Emotions

"TODAY IS ON HOLD"

My normal routines, the responsibilities,
that I do without a second thought,
has been put on a temporary hold,
in limbo and so lost.
I do not know how long I'll be away,
I hope not until I'm old.
My impatience gets the best of me,
don't let this take too long.

Who will do the things that I need to have done,
will someone be there for me,
I have a worry that my old life,
will lose its responsibilities.
The need for money, to feel my worth,
is trying to leave me now,
so how will I be able to work on through,
the things that make me scowl.

My life's uncertain, it is going to change,
those things in my past just was,
will all get done so differently
and go on as it always has.
I will trust the people in my life,
to take over and help me out,
and work on just the things I need,
to make me come about.

Today is on hold, of the things that I,
did just a short while ago,
I need to allow my life today,
to be healthy so I can grow.
Responsibilities come in many ways,
but most importantly,
I have to do the healthy ones,
to have a life with me.

It's OK my past's on hold,
those things I knew so well,
I have a new direction now,
with responsibilities that I can tell.
So helpers please just do what you can,
to keep my past alive, and I will do the things today,
to be sure I will survive.

Personal Emotions

"WITHIN MY SOUL"

My feelings inside move around me so,
they bring joys and tears to me.
I know I am still so alive today,
but with so much painful uncertainty.
I try to get inside my soul, inside that part of me,
that brings me back to that special place,
where I just need to try to be.

Within my soul, that place called home,
that keeps me moving up,
This special feeling I can remember,
I keep close, and never give up.
The loneliness, the fear of pain,
combines within my soul,
and has me thinking about my future,
no guarantees for my home.

I need to understand the feeling of pain,
its swirling uncertainty,
and try to bring it into my thoughts,
to feel my true reality.
The feelings will always be with me, to analyze my past,
but I just need to see today,
as my helpful looking glass.

Within my soul there is a strength,
that has the power to conquer what lies ahead,
I just need to keep myself together,
and deal with all the bad.
So as I look at every day that tests my inner soul,
I will look into the eye of the storm
and not let it take its hold.

Personal Emotions

"ALL CHOICES ARE MINE"

To plan my future, the choice is clear,
determine the action to take,
and understand the consequences of mistakes,
without a long debate.
I know there are no guarantees,
or a way to foresee my plans,
but all the choices I make today,
will be how I make my stand.

For all the choices to be mine,
does not mean advice is not desired,
but understanding from you all,
will make me feel less tired.
I want the best for my life, I want to live so long,
but all these choices have to be mine,
so I can carry on.

I fear for pain, for loneliness too,
the uncertainty drives me mad,
I hope that you just understand
and will not be too awfully sad.
I am the same as I was before,
and even after the choice is made,
I will be with you all the time,
who I am will never fade.

I know the optimism for my future, I see what I want to do,
I just want after all my decisions,
that you will be there too.
So give support, your opinions please, with all the love you can,
but I will make my final decision,
to live as who I am.

Personal Emotions

"A LOVER'S PRAYER"

When you are touched by an angel, heaven opens up,
to show you a wonderful world,
the life I have is more beautiful,
with you as my wonderful girl.
The rays from your face always brightens up,
whatever tries to make ill of my mood,
I appreciate all that you give to me,
it should be understood.

Today I see a different face,
the rays not as bright as they were,
the pain inside is too easy to see,
as you attempt to keep it blurred.
I want to take inside of me
the fear you seem to have,
and take control of all the pain,
to free you from being sad.

I will always be there to help you move,
through the days of fear and pain,
with love for you that I hope will help,
to bring you relief once again.
I pray each day that I might awake
and be the one in this awful pain,
it is my only wish for you,
to be back just whole again.

Alone you're not, or going to need,
to concern yourself with worry,
as I will take upon myself to be
the new responsible party.
The things that you are worrying about
and the things that make you cry,
will be the duties I take on,
while you work to stay alive.

Personal Emotions

"WILL I REMEMBER MY PRECIOUS MOMENTS?"

Before the news, my moments went by, without a care in the world.
I took each day with gratitude that I could always unfurl.
Today my life is affected with, the mystery of many unknowns,
my precious moments that I once had, seem to be so all alone.

The past for me does bring me smiles, I felt my life was good,
but now I think that time is short, my feelings are so confused.
Will I remember my precious moments, or will they fade away,
so I might live with all my pain and the fear I have each day.

I need to think that my new life, will build new memories,
if only I can stay away from all the negative uncertainties.
It is too easy to dwell and ponder, on all the negative thoughts
I have, but it does not make getting through the reality that
I feel is awfully bad.

I have to try to remember me, with all my triumphs past, and use
the precious moments they were, to make today just last.
I am still me, just some change inside that should make me stop
and think, that today is the beginning of New Precious Moments
that I just need to link.

I will remember my precious moments, but not just as my past,
and continue being who I am so my new precious moments will
always last.

Personal Emotions

"BUILDING MY MINDSET"

Each day that I learn more about my disease,
each day that I gain additional facts,
each day it gets more confusing to me,
so I'm planning my Mindset Attack.

The information that I have, will be used to mark the course
of action I take, I need to just go with the decisions that show,
and won't make my mindset ache.
This is my life that I know is at stake, so a decision is needed by me,
it will be one that is good, and the best that it could be.

I know that many have gone before me,
And many have survived quite well,
But how do I know what decision to take,
That will not put me in a living hell.

Should I go with the odds, the proven results,
and just make sure I kill those ugly cells, and get on with my life,
without stress or unneeded strife,
to be part of the world I love so well.

Building my Mindset is not easy to do,
I get confused everyday that I read,
and it only brings up much unwanted disgust,
and not allowing a decision to be.

The last of the tests are upon me now,
and the decision is coming to a head,
so my mindset must be prepared, to be ready or be sad.
I can decide the right course I should take, Or let others decide for me.
I just need to do what is best for my life, So I'll be around for all to see.

There are no right or wrong answers to choose,
Just making them gives me the fits.
I'll close my eyes and pray I'm right
and trust my internal wits.

Personal Emotions

_____
_____
_____
_____
_____
_____
_____
_____
_____
_____
_____
_____
_____
_____
_____
_____
_____
_____
_____
_____
_____
_____
_____
_____

"I AM IN CONTROL"

No matter the news or the problems that arise,
I will always be in control.
My destiny is set by the powers that be,
but, I am in control.

How goes my life today or tomorrow,
is not governed by things of my past,
my future is set by the controls that I place,
on my actions that make my life a blast.

Each day will have set backs,
or problems that will appear,
I will keep to my long range plans,
and not let the detours of life's normal hurdles,
disrupt or not allow me to stand.

Today I could receive the greatest of news,
maybe tomorrow the news won't fair so well,
but what has to be, is a force inside me,
that tells me that all in my life will be swell.

I am in control and will always be,
no matter what crosses my path,
everyday I am here,
I will go through every year,
living my life as if it were my last.

Personal Emotions

_____
_____
_____
_____
_____
_____
_____
_____
_____
_____
_____
_____
_____
_____
_____
_____
_____
_____
_____
_____

"BELIEVE IN MY LIFE"

It takes just a moment to change your life,
from the normal things you do everyday.
Your life can be fragile with unfortunate news,
that can carry your plans away.

Today you can't believe in a life that you had,
that would take you through the end of your years,
and now you have news that can change what you do,
with beliefs that combine with your fears.

To believe in your life, should not be governed,
by the health or the state that you're in,
but should keep to its purpose,
with beliefs that are curious,
to enjoy your life from within.

So believe in your life,
it is there just for you,
no matter the direction it takes,
and stand very tall,
and grab on to it all,
and enjoy it with laughter and cheers.

Personal Emotions

"AM I REALLY CURED?"

The tests are over, the results are in,
the course of action is set, but will this all be
the cure that's right for me, I continue to hope for the best.
The positive answer is "we don't know, but it appears
your cells are behaving", I just keep the faith of what they say,
to keep me from going crazy.

Am I really cured? I will never know,
I will always be on the alert. I'll watch earnestly,
for any symptoms that I can see,
that might bring back the painful hurt.
My life has changed the way I think,
the way I feel and move, I have to keep my attitude in,
a state of positive mood.

I continue to hear some glowing reports of others who beat the odds,
but what sticks in my mind to drive me insane,
are the stories of the ones who lost.
Will this be me the one who will, find out that all the cells have spread,
or will I just be the one who goes on without worry,
that won't keep me lying in my bed.

The cure for me just has to be, the attitude that I make,
to not allow this disease, to take over and control me,
and hurt me and make me break.
I will never know if I am really cured,
or if the cells inside me are dead.
But keeping myself with an attitude that's right,
should keep me out of bed.

I will go on after all the tests, after all the action I take,
and keep my life just as it was, this is my cure that is at stake.
I am the one who will cure me now, and keep me from any more pain,
and live my life in the world I choose, this is the promise that I make.

Personal Emotions

"FRIENDSHIP WORDS"

The people I know express their emotions,
to let me know they care.
Each of them uncomfortable with their feelings,
I shudder at all of their despair.
But nonetheless, I love their words,
their care for me right now.
It is a helping hand to know,
that they are there and will be around.

I take each word, each phrase I hear,
and listen with my friendship heart.
And shed a tear to let them know,
I feel their emotional part.
I can not convince them, I'll be ok,
or that this disease will be cured right now.
But all I can offer is my pledge to them,
that I plan to be around.

I am so rich, a wealth of sorts,
that is only measured by who is near.
These are my personal possessions I have,
that will keep me moving through all my years.
I measure my life, just by who I am,
by the people I call my friends,
and treasure all their friendship words,
over and over again.

Personal Emotions

"LISTEN REAL HARD"

As each day moves forward, with tests that exhausts,
just try to listen as your body speaks.
Open your mind to the results you need to know,
no negative thoughts should leak.
Don't focus on the pain you feel this day,
or the tired way you move,
but listen real hard to the message inside,
that is there to be understood.

These next weeks, the months you take,
to fight to defeat those cells,
requires that you keep to your plan,
with an attitude that will begin to grow and swell.
No matter the tests or the way you feel,
should make you turn away,
from the only goal you have right now,
to stay alive and ready to play.

The helpers you have are there to guide,
to keep you in your fold
and offer advice that is to help you defeat,
and achieve your needed goals.
So listen real hard to what is said,
and to what is in your heart,
this attitude will help you through,
the most upcoming difficult parts.

It's only you that can complete this task,
to fight for what you want,
to keep to the suggested plan you have,
without faltering or falling apart.
You need to continue to listen real hard,
to follow the directions you have,
and you will in a short, short while,
have your victory over all that is bad.

Personal Emotions

_____
_____
_____
_____
_____
_____
_____
_____
_____
_____
_____
_____
_____
_____
_____
_____
_____
_____
_____
_____
_____
_____
_____

"CONFUSED CELLS"

It's time to rename the most horrible word, the word that describes a death to you. It has a meaning that forms a picture, that destroys the hope that's true.

When you hear the word CANCER, a chill forms inside, bringing tears, and fears to all who are around. This word has an affect that can cause you to cry, and make the most controlled person come tumbling down.

So why put a name on your condition, when first it is detected for you, it causes your mind to imagine the worst when this condition might not be so true. The word, the phrase, it's such a horrible state, to have your mind fall into the blues, especially because your doctors are not sure what stage your cells are in too.

I propose to begin with a correct group of words, that describes the beginning for you, it will allow you to adjust to the state that you're in, including the people around who love you.

"Confused Cells" are the words that we need, to call the first stage that we're in, it has a meaning that instantly tells you, that there's tests and work to begin. Cancer when heard, is a tattoo you will have, that will never be fully removed, but Confused Cells when heard from the start, will not allow you to be confused.

*So it's time to rename this unfortunate word,
with two words that describes what you have,
and to remove from your brain,
that bad word with its pain,
and begin to come out of the dark.*

Personal Emotions

"INTERNAL HEALING FLAME"

We have a control valve inside our bodies,
that has the power to hurt or heal.
The flame burns all the time very low,
and most of all concealed.
To heal your body requires that this flame be hot as coal,
to burn away all the problems you face,
that are deep within our souls.

The flame burns hot when you laugh real hard,
or when you feel real love.
You feel your body just has such release,
feeling the magic from above.
But, when you let your emotions rule,
the way your mood should go,
the flame becomes so very cold,
allowing the problems to grow.

To keep your flame burning hot, requires a lot to do,
to keep your smiles with laughter coming,
from deep inside of you.
Go find somewhere to laugh real hard
or be with someone that cares
and keep your positive attitude burning,
and climb those successful stairs.

Stay away from all the negative sounds,
or the people who bring you down,
and find the place where you can have,
all the positive wonderful sounds.
So as you go through everyday,
be sure you have with you, the needed Internal Healing Flame,
that will keep all your problems away from you.

Personal Emotions

"YOUR EARTH MOTHER"

It's all around, a protective force, that is there to sustain your life.
It is so natural that we at times, do not believe it's right.
There is a reason that our world,
was created the way it was,
we just have to understand what there is to use,
its powers are sent from above.

We tend to think that commercial finds, are promised results for life.
Are the only things that are good for us, to help us with our fights.
But, there are so many natural things,
when used in its proper way,
will brings us back to Mother Earth,
to nurture us in many ways.

We give the plants, the trees, our life, they return it back with no fuss,
so why don't we accept that they, are the medicine for all of us?
The plants, the trees create the air,
we all take so naturally,
let's continue taking other things they have,
to help our misery.

I don't believe that all chemicals, are natural for us to take,
I want to let the things of earth, come back to me each day.
It can not hurt or harm me now,
my Mother Earth is right,
to help me each and everyday,
to build a healthy life.

I will give to you, the earth I love, the part of life you need,
and I will allow you to pay me back, with the medicine you have for me.
As we become in harmony,
each day that I'm around,
I will treasure all you have to give,
that will make my life so sound.

Personal Emotions

_____
_____
_____
_____
_____
_____
_____
_____
_____
_____
_____
_____
_____
_____
_____
_____
_____
_____
_____
_____
_____
_____

"I FEEL YOUR TEARS"

Don't hide from me, the tears you have,
or hide the fear inside,
I feel your tears each day I'm near,
they are no unknown surprise.
Each tear you shed is caught by me,
in a pouch inside my heart,
I use it to fuel my love for you,
to build a wonderful part.

When first you promised to be with me,
for the lifetime that you have,
I committed to be with you through the times that were so sad.
We are a team that will succeed and complete our lifetime goals,
so please don't hide your tears from me,
they help my life unfold.

You need to let me feel your tears,
just let them leave your heart,
and I will use them to give you back,
a love that is not dark.
To hide your tears, with fears locked up,
inside that soul you have,
will shut me out, from who you are,
and make me feel so bad.

My life is yours, like yours is mine,
don't hide a thing from me,
I have to be so close to you, to help you through this breeze.
We are just as one, a bond that's made from a love we both give out,
so please let me feel your tears,
I understand what it's all about.

Personal Emotions

"UNCONTROLLED MOODS"

Before the news, that changed your life,
your moods came from a different place,
and now they take on a different mode,
to keep you in a confused state.
It's alright to go, with your moods, as uncontrolled as they might seem,
it's how your heart is dealing with, this most terrifying horrible thing.

You have a label, a mark of sorts,
that won't allow you to be what you were,
so let the uncontrolled moods you have,
open other, different doors.
Your life is changed, you can not remove, the thoughts inside your head,
so don't frustrate your heart each day thinking that you are almost dead.

Death will come when your time is up,
it can't be foreseen today,
so let your moods just flow with you,
to keep your life at play.
Take time to reflect on what you want, in the life you see right now,
and live it to its fullest level, with no regrets, and no facial scowls.

Let the uncontrolled moods you have,
be actions that bring new life to you,
and create a time that has you doing,
all the things you want to do.
Be spontaneous, each day you have, appreciate what your day offers you,
and see the uncontrolled moods you have, turn out to not be blue.

Share these moods with all your friends,
to teach them all about your life,
and help them see the person you are, and how you get through strife.
Your moods are yours, it's understood,
they will change each day that you're here,
so why not make them be so very beautiful,
each and every year.

Personal Emotions

"THE GRIM WEEPER"

Are you the type who cries at will,
to make your point too clear?
or do you do it for the attention,
to bring everyone too near?
Are you a Grim Weeper who cries at things,
that others would just not do?
Is crying how you express yourself,
to get what's right for you?

The Grim Weeper is in all of us if we let ourselves be loose,
but is it how to conquer fear and all the unpleasant things we do.
To weep or cry should come from a place,
that is deep within your soul,
and should only be for you alone,
to treasure and to hold.

So when you feel the urge to cry,
to weep about your pain,
be sure you weep just for you,
without control or passing blame.
It is ok to cry and weep for all you're going through,
but make sure that you cry and weep real hard,
to defeat your trouble too.

Be a fighter, with a mind so strong,
that makes you conquer and defeat,
with tears of anger that you show, that keeps you on your feet.
To be a Grim Weeper only makes for you,
a weakness for you to bail,
but weeping with a strength inside,
will not allow you to fail.

Personal Emotions

"AN END FOR A BEGINNING"

For me it's relief, the final test will come,
and I will move on to the cure,
my new life has begun.
I have this hope that's just for me,
the results I see them clear,
that I will defeat this Cancer inside,
And not let it stay so near.

Is there doubt inside, this confused mind I have,
that has the power to knock me down,
or do I have still left inside,
the strength to move around.

I believe this is a beginning,
a new one that's just for me,
to set my course for my life to come,
with hope and harmony.
I will plan each day with courage that's strong,
and fight to save my life,
I won't allow this fear inside
to wreak havoc on my life.

This will be an end to a horrible time,
a new beginning with plans and goals.
I will feel such emotional relief,
when the final results are told.

So as I close this final chapter on the tests that put fear in me,
I will handle the next fight just the same
without falling to my knees.
With strength and fortitude I will win out during this horrible time,
and put an end to all my fears,
with a new beginning that's ready to shine.

Personal Emotions

"THE WHISPERING LOVE CHANT"

It comes around, in a low soft sound,
the words that bring life to our souls,
it is a welcome voice we hear,
even when we're away all alone.
A whispering love chant, the words that tell,
of how you are seen by your mate,
the words are clear, and oh so dear,
to make your life so great.

Sometimes the words are kept away,
to bring out a future feel,
but no matter how long it's been, the feelings remain so real.
To chant your love to someone special,
is a gift beyond compare,
and it will bring big dividends,
as your relationship moves on in years.

So when you feel the urge to chant,
those special whispering words,
be open with your feelings each time,
to express your total worth.
There is no rule or time that's best, to express just how you feel,
just do it when you need to tell,
your lover just how your loves for real.

The Whispering Love Chant is for everyone,
it just needs to get out each time, to tell the person in your life,
that your life with them is just so fine.
So say it clear, without holding back,
just how deep your feelings go,
and say it with the honesty,
that will show your inner glow.

Personal Emotions

"WHO WILL I BE?"

This life I had some months ago,
was changed in a sudden rage,
I was given a new role to project,
that changed the way I play.
I didn't know if I was to be,
the death that was supposed to come late in life,
or was I to become some victim,
or someone who had a nasty fight.

Who will I be, as my days roll on with tests that try my soul,
it's coming to a head right now,
which way I am supposed to go.
Have I decided who I want to be or am I still the same,
it's hard to know just who I am,
since getting my new name.

I know that everyone in my life,
wishes that I will be just ok,
and get through all of this real soon,
and go back to similar ways.
But, I am just too torn to know just who I want to be,
I have this great new change that's there,
I am curious, so I must see.

Who will I be, as these days roll by,
and the months turn into years,
I know I will not be the same that was,
I am mixed with too many fears.
I hope I take with me today,
the person that I love,
and blend it with the person I've become,
to find my new fitting gloves.

Personal Emotions

_____

_____

_____

_____

_____

_____

_____

_____

_____

_____

_____

_____

_____

_____

_____

_____

_____

_____

_____

_____

_____

_____

"FRIENDSHIP FIRST, LOVER SECOND"

The biggest fear I have inside, is can I be there for you?
I have never been in a situation like this to test me through and through.
I was your friend when first we made our decision to bond real tight,
I kept this friendship in my heart, it made my love just right.

Today I have a role to play, the support that is needed for you,
I am a little scared right now of not knowing just what to do.
Its easy to talk and act with care, when problems are not so great,
but will I be able to be there for you, will I step up to the plate?

I love you so, you mean more to me, than anything in this life,
I want to be there just for you, and squeeze you oh so tight.
I have to think and instill a friendship kind of attitude,
and change my thoughts from lover first, this has to be understood.

I will attempt to be your friend, to mix it with who I am,
and be the lover that you need, with a warm outstretched powerful hand.
Don't try to attempt to do for you, these days of needed help,
I have the strength and desire to be a rock that once was felt.

I have the experience to handle things, that most will run from fast,
and be the one who's there for you, with love that will forever last.
So just plan your days of recouping your strength,
don't think you have much to do, I will be there as your friend each day,
and as your lover too.

Personal Emotions

Personal Emotions

Personal Emotions

Part Three
WHAT HAPPENS NEXT?

You've struggled for answers up to this point, being honest and truthful to yourself. It is possible, however, that the answers that have come out, through the expression of your emotions, are still cloudy and uncertain. Getting to this point in the book is a good indication that you are letting out the fear and loneliness you keep feeling before you started reading this book.

So what happens next? You continue to keep journaling your emotions in the Mind Diet way to keep strengthening your resolve. The next grouping of poems should touch a different part of you, allowing the release of feelings that have not come out before.

There is a certain "darkness," I've been told by other cancer survivors, that never seems to leave. It is like a bad dream that never goes away; the fear of your cancer returning. Now, more than ever, you should put your fears and hopelessness onto paper. Find that special rhythm inside your heart that will help you move forward into a shinning light of hope and happiness. Delegate your worst feelings and emotions to your rhythm poetry and get it out of your head so you can see the life you have around you and experience all the Mind Diets you deserve.

The first poem in this section was inspired by my fear that I might lose my wife, Nancy, to cancer. I realized I had no control over what was going on in her body and scared that I could not be with her during her operation.

To add to my fear and sadness, was the worry from our best friend, Anita and my mother. Both of them loved her as much as I love her, but from their own place in their heart.

"The Spirit Stone," (four separate pieces) a special blown glass paper-weight, was held in our hands in order to stay connected to Nancy with our thoughts. Nancy had held each of them prior to her operation so her energy would be transferred to the three of us. I gave her my own "Spirit Stone" so she could have my strength and love while she went under the knife.

I believe that a part of the person remains on the Spirit Stone, and gets transferred to the person who needs our prayers in this case it was Nancy.

Nancy and I have used the Spirit Stone during the numerous heart procedures I had to go through since 1999. Just knowing I had a part of Nancy with me during a scary time made the ordeal bearable.

The Poem "Spirit Friend" communicates a special love I have toward my wife. I hope you can find a Spirit Friend in your life.

I've tried to create the next group of poems as a way to open up a floodgate of emotions. So be prepared. Remember, be honest and truthful and you will get through this unbearable time.

"THE SPIRIT FRIEND"

Our souls are connected by the thoughts we have,
when we think of the people we love.
The connection runs deep, our spirit flies high,
with the chants as our heart gives its beat.

The spirit connects as we touch and think,
of the times when our friendship was high,
and the spirit soars greater,
when we hold in our hands,
something of the person we just love all the time.

A blessing is made with this stone made of glass,
from the earth, which we all first called home,
and the touch that we make, will be our bond that can't break,
as we think of the one our love is for.

A friendship is something that tests who we are,
when the times place a challenge in our way,
and this stone brings to us, the people who we trust,
in our hearts and our souls everyday.

When you need to connect with the person that you love,
be sure to hold tight this spirit stone,
and watch how you'll see the magic that can be,
when the spirit friend comes into your home.

Personal Emotions

"SURVIVAL IS A CHOICE"

Everything that is, that's in your life,
is a choice that comes from you,
the way you live your life each day, tells the world so much that's true.
There is no fate, or luck that is, the controlling force of you,
but just the choice you make each day,
to live your life in view.

Each day we awake to make a choice,
that takes us down our road,
the choice is so important each time, it builds upon things we hold.
Survival comes, from what we want, each moment that we're here,
and molds itself to form the image,
of what we care to bear.

Its how we choose to define our self,
with our attitude towards the world,
that makes the way we survive each day, to participate and unfurl.
So never think that life just is, or that luck needs to come only to you,
just understand that survival comes,
as a choice that is from the truth.

So when your life seems just too bleak,
or not as you want it to be,
take a good look at what you are, and the choices you need to see.
If you just want to change your life, the choice is up to you,
it needs to hear, from deep inside,
that this is really what you want it to do.

Each day the test comes to you clear,
of how to survive today, its attitude, with eyes so true,
that makes you do the things that work your way.
Don't ever give up, or think you're done, when life seems hard to bear,
just lift your head up to the sky,
the good choices are very clear.

Personal Emotions

"WAITING WITH MY GHOSTS"

Each moment I'm alone, the ghosts arrive ,
they're always a determined group,
injecting a negative power, to control and disrupt my moods.
They crawl inside your head each day,
instilling their fearful attitude,
with all the intent of controlling your outlook,
with a negative, defeating mood.

Why they come or why they stay,
can be a mystery if left unchecked,
they seem to want to make a life, seem dreadful and a wreck.
They serve no purpose or contribute to life,
a meaningful solution for you,
they need to be kicked out of your head,
before their damage begins to brew.

Each time they appear, you let them in,
but with a smile so big and bright,
and give them back your thoughts of love,
and that you're ready for a fight.
If you're determined to kick them out,
then watch their faces turn white,
and see them leave you in a big bad huff,
never again you'll feel the fright.

It only took a moment,
but they left without a good-bye,
to leave you once again alone,
your thoughts right by your side.
Just lean on back and smile real big,
you have a chance to win,
the game of solving all your problems,
that control comes from within.

Personal Emotions

"I'M READY, BRING ON THE FIGHT"

Since round one began, I hit the mat,
I almost got knocked out too quick,
but I got up and began to fight back,
and made my punches stick.
Each round I'm in, I appear to win,
the fight is going my way,
so keep the challenges coming at me,
I will make them fade away.

The fear I had, has turned to rage,
with energy to save my life,
I know the course I'm going to take,
to win this nasty fight.
Each test I take, I win real fast,
so what's in store for me?
I am so ready to take it all on,
but are you prepared for what you'll see?

As days move on I'll get real strong,
the tests will be over for me,
and I will just be set to make,
the life that is meant to be.
So hear me now, I'm ready for you,
bring on the best fight you have,
I will defeat you with all my heart,
because I'm very mad.

Personal Emotions

"I CAN'T FAIL"

I knew before what friends I had, I never doubted their love,
but now they are right there with me,
with support like a good fitting glove.
My heart beats fast, my emotions fly high,
their words bring tears to me,
I cannot fail, when they're by my side,
this fact is so plain to see.

There is no fail in my attitude, as time will tell its tale,
I only want to move real fast, to end this time in jail.
I will not get defeated,
though hard work lays ahead,
I'll keep my body moving each day,
and keep it out of bed.

My course is set to conquer this disease, there is no compromise,
I will only accept a total win, as my final winning prize.
With all my friends right by my side,
with their words of love for me,
I can not fail no matter what,
their power encourages me.

From Can't to Won't, to Win, to Success,
will be words that stay in my head,
and each day as I work real hard,
there will be no other words instead.
I can't fail, I see it now, I have this disease running scared,
I will each day, keep my head on straight,
I know I cannot fail!

Personal Emotions

"YOU SAID WHAT?

So many instructions to file in my head, it is whirling just so fast,
From draining my pump, to loosening my stool,
won't they ever begin to let up?
The pills have their rules, that need recording each time,
so I won't trip through my days in a fog,
but wait, did they say it's ok to goof up,
with the pills or the pump with the jar?
I am not as young as I used to be, I need to write everything down,
if this is the trend of the instructions to come,
then how many forests will I bring down.
It will go by fast, the healing I need,
as I begin the most important job for me,
to kill all those cells that are inside of my body,
trying to find a path for their greed.

You said what? Please repeat that last comment!
six weeks, everyday for my burn?
Will I remember to go, as my body begins to slow,
from the cure that is supposed to not allow the cells to return?
So understand this, as you dictate my instructions,
I want to follow all that you want me to do,
but please understand, that my head just can stand,
only so many things, that you continue to put me through.

I will lose my patience, with all who's around,
from the doctors, to my lover at first,
but please bear in mind that it is not personal every time,
that I appear to be angry at you.
I will do all I can, on my own as I stand,
ready to fight this disgusting disease, but be ready anytime,
I might need your help at times, to interpret the things I must do.
"You said What?" You understand me,
and you love me just the way that I am, so let's all just go,
through these instructions very slow,
so I can show you that I truly understand.

Personal Emotions

"I FEEL GREAT"

Is it all true, what they say I have, and what is in store for me?
I feel so good and healthy inside, I am confused as I can be.
Since my first test, that found the cells, that placed a mark on my soul,
now the remaining tests have proved all negative,
am I done, can I begin to unfold?

I have been cut, with parts removed, now twice, to end my tests,
so why do I continue to feel, again so at my best.
Is this all real, or some bad dream,
that I will awake from real soon, or am I just so organized,
that I found this problem at its first bloom?

I can't sit down or relax too long, it's not who I want to be,
but I know I must relax right now, the hard work comes soon to me.
I'll take advantage of all this time, to allow the care I need,
I am so happy that all is great, as I defeat this terrible disease.

It's just organize, a little here, and put things in their place,
I feel the strength to do it all, I'm at my normal pace.
I hear the yells to relax right now, and let others do for me,
but I just need a little more time, to believe in what I see.

I promise this, that I will soon, be a patient who's relaxing well,
and let you all take care of me, through this stressful living hell.
But if I break my promise to you, just smile at me each time,
it's just that I might not feel ok about resting all the time.

I feel just great, I want you all, to understand this stressful time,
I will be doing as much as I can, this attitude keeps me fine.
So catch me doing the my normal things, and scold me if you must,
but I feel great at what I'm doing, so what is all the fuss?

Personal Emotions

" A LOVER'S FLAME"

For many years you gave me love, today is just the same,
the level I feel that comes from your heart,
continues to burn its warm flame.
But now I need to give back to you,
what you have given each day to me,
to help you through this time of worry,
It's oh so necessary.

This love has been growing deep inside,
and nurtured each day by you,
to make the act of giving you love,
the easiest thing to do.
I want you to just relax and enjoy,
the care that will come your way,
this is my lover's wish to you,
to bring you some sunny days.

There is no effort or energy,
that I need to have ready for you,
the feelings of my love inside,
is all that I need to get me through.
Don't think you're a burden,
or that you will bother me just too much,
I owe you more than I can give,
I can never payback enough.

So please take this Lover's Wish, to be healthy and live quite long,
I will be right by your side, helping you to remain so very strong.
There is no measure of what I can do, I know you'd do the same,
so please sit back and just relax, and enjoy this lover's flame.

Personal Emotions

"LETS GET GOING"

I'm ready now to begin my work,
I don't want to wait any longer,
I have this desire to destroy those nasty cells,
before they begin to loiter.

Let's get going to rid me of this,
that terrible word called Cancer,
I am so impatient I can't hold back,
this is, my only answer.

No matter the pain, or the time it will take,
I just want to get on with this chore,
and fight so very hard for me,
against this thing that I deplore.

I am not scared or frightened now,
as I have them on the run,
I will take no prisoners,
as I move toward my new life,
that has just begun.

So let's get going, I am in a groove,
each challenge for me is that's there,
is going to be defeated with ease,
this is what I now declare!

Personal Emotions

"PAINT A PICTURE"

Your life is images that you paint,
with colors that make you feel good,
the scenes you have inside your head,
give encouragement as it should.
Each day your challenges attempt to form, new images in your mind,
you need to keep your happy scenes,
with the brightest colors you can find.

There are those days, that dark colors appear,
on the palette you call your life,
to try to change the picture you have,
to cause some inner fights.
But you must always add the colors,
that paint the scenes you like,
and never paint a picture each day,
until you get the colors right.

As the days will come that are just so dark,
they will leave you just as fast,
you have to mix your colors right,
to create the scenes that will last.
But keep in mind that the painted picture, you have inside your head,
comes only from the scenes you want,
that keeps you out of bed.

So paint the picture of what you want,
make it as bright as it can be,
and never let those dark, dark days,
take over what you see.
It's up to you, it always is,
so focus on what you need,
and don't let any challenges you face,
paint a picture you don't want to see.

Personal Emotions

"LITTLE STEPS"

The natural effort is to jump right in,
to begin to improve your wounds,
but little steps are needed now,
that will make your progress bloom.
Impatience will need to be controlled by you,
at every move you make,
to insure you take to the final test,
without making any mistakes.

Take little steps that make you move,
always forward, toward your goal,
take little steps each time,
you try to improve your present hold.
Don't rush because you have a goal,
or a time table that's pressuring you,
your little steps will get you there,
on time so your life will resume.

All things you'll do throughout this time,
will move at its own pace,
and let you get to your goal on time,
and completed to keep you in your race.
Little Steps, add up to steps,
that will accumulate into to large,
and you will see that what you've done,
is the best you could by far.

Personal Emotions

"A SPECIAL TIRED"

My eyes are beginning to close,
they signal my rest is needed,
I want to continue to participate some more,
but my energy is almost depleted.
A little rest is all I need,
to get back in the world again,
my strength will come back to me so normal,
so I can fight harder and harder again.

This is a special kind of tired,
a place where healing is formed,
it needs to be nurtured in such a way,
to make me become so very strong.
I do not like or even enjoy,
this slow down I have with me,
but I will wait for just a while,
and let everything just hover and be.

I will appreciate this time I have,
to reflect on who I am,
I will not allow this tired feeling to overwhelm,
and make me feel so damned.
A special tired that I feel,
tells me my life is beginning,
but all I need is a little time,
to make it now so wonderfully fitting.

Personal Emotions

"HELPERS AFOOT"

Which ever way you look,
there are helpers there for you,
their job is to only care and assist.
You need to let them be,
as uncomfortable as you are,
so they can keep you out of the pits.

No matter what they do,
it's with love for you each time,
with the goal to get you to a healthy point,
and then turn it over to you, so you can shine.

A helper has a heart of gold,
that comes from a scared part,
to help them fulfill a true desire,
to your broken parts.

So just sit back awhile,
enjoy this time you have,
to reflect and heal your loving soul,
and let the helpers do,
all that they really want for you,
to be part of your life right now in style.

Personal Emotions

"WORTHLESS FEELINGS"

I feel like I am a troubled person, fighting hard within myself,
not knowing who or what I'll be, my mind fights with itself.
These feelings come from all the pain I have,
that makes me think how worthless I must seem,
and make me walk on egg shells each day,
my moods have such negative swings.

From lack of energy, to too much pain, my mind goes to its darkest place,
I fight the tears that build inside, causing me to think this is my fate.
I never before depended on others, to help me out at times,
but now I must rely on them, it's a terrible way to shine.

These worthless feelings are known to me, to be figments of my mind,
but I just can't remove them fast, to find some precious time.
My emotions build in such a way, that my energy is drained so much,
that I continue to think I am not worthy of even a touch.

I need to think each time I feel, unworthy and in the pits,
and see the people all around, who see the worth in me that is.
The pain, the drugs, and inactivity, contribute to my inner toil,
so I must look the other way, and not let my emotions stay,
in a continued slow boil.

When I begin to go into those Worthless Feeling Moods,
I need to look all around, to see a better attitude.
It's me that needs to learn just how, to control these feelings inside,
and reach inside my wonderful self and pull out my worthy pride.

This time is temporary, and will soon pass,
these feeling will be gone real soon,
and I will find that these worthless feelings, just didn't need to bloom.
I will begin to be active again, to exercise my pain away,
and get back all the energy I had,
that will keep all the worthless feelings away.

Personal Emotions

"SWIMMING IN YOUR FRAGILE SOUL"

How you feel, or how you worry,
is shared by me right now,
I come from a different place than you,
your soul is mine for now.
Each day I try to swim in the currents,
of your fragile delicate soul,
to try to rescue what I can,
to help you become again whole.

I am your lifeguard, that watches you,
to support your every move,
and will jump right in to help you swim,
through the rip tides you're going through.
I will not panic or rush too fast,
when I see you struggle through your maze,
but will be there with help so near,
during these important troubled days.

I like to swim inside your soul,
during calm or stormy times,
I am just there to love you so,
and make your place just mine.
This time for me, is difficult,
to see you as weak as you are,
but I will swim right by your side,
with support and love not far.

So as you continue to swim each day,
through the tides and currents of your soul,
just understand, I have a hand,
so you know you're not alone.

Personal Emotions

"WILL I STILL BE PRETTY?"

What I was, is gone for good,
a new person is forming inside.
Will I be as pretty as before?
I can't deal with one more surprise.

Part of my body has changed from a knife,
other parts have changed by thoughts,
but all I want is to be the person,
who will not ever become lost.

Will I ever be 100%,
or will I remain a fragile wreck,
I just want to go back again,
to the time before this event.

I see my face, its lines just speak,
of the emotions inside of my head,
but I still see the person I knew back when,
I bounced right off my bed.

Can I be as pretty as before,
from the inside to my other skin,
and have a life that makes me feel,
as pretty as I once had been.

If all it takes is to change my thoughts,
to bring out the beauty in me,
then I will act as pretty as I can,
and be as happy as everyone can see.

Will I be as pretty as before,
I think that choice has been made.
My life has changed with no return,
My reflection is carved in stone,
I see a new beauty inside to treasure and to hold.

Will I be pretty, oh yes I will,
come see the new improved me,
my smiles and energy that I show,
is all the beauty that I need.

Personal Emotions

"APPRECIATED PROGRESS"

I thought I would be worse off than I am,
with pain that would keep me in bed,
I worried so much that I didn't believe,
all the encouragement around that was said.

It has only been a short period of time,
and look how well I can do,
my progress is going much faster than I thought,
this I, appreciate too.

I still have an energy loss,
with pain that makes me so scared,
but each day my progress gets better for me,
I am not feeling as once I had.

Impatience can take all the effort that I made,
and convince me that progress is slow,
but reality shows that my progress has grown,
way ahead of where it should go.

Appreciate my progress,
that's what I should say to me,
and see the improvement that I've made,
it is my reality.

I need to remember that it has been a short time,
that I started to make my move,
so I won't get depressed if I still feel a mess,
my progress is in a groove.

So appreciate all that you've done,
take the good with all the bad,
and keep on working hard each day,
and appreciate what you have.

Personal Emotions

"WHAT'S MY SCORE"

Evaluation is hard for me, as the pain just hurts so much,
it seemed so different than the other day,
I feel like giving up.
I can't remember those beginning days,
when my fear mixed with the pain,
so how can I evaluate,
each day just seems the same.

At night it appears to be intense, while I am alone in my inner world,
It goes by at a turtle's pace,
as my life begins to unfurl.
The morning comes, I feel the tiredness,
of my night-time episodes,
and wonder if today will be a set-back,
that will begin to unfold.

Let's take a look at where you were, in your pain and fear before,
and place a score upon it now,
to compare for evermore.
Now what's your score, this day you have,
to compare just how you feel,
I think you'll find an impressive score,
that is ready to reveal.

Don't mix your feelings of healing you have,
with the beginning pain that was there,
and be as honest as you can,
and place a score that's fair.
There is improvement, from pain and thoughts,
you know you must have hope,
but you just need this all to be over,
this unfortunate, ugly joke.

Personal Emotions

"FEELINGS"

Each moment that is with me today,
moves in many new directions,
causing confusion of sorts for me,
and many apprehensions.
These feelings come from a place inside,
that is not a comfort or support,
I have these crazy feelings inside,
it affects my inner worth.

I worry about being whole again ,
and back to my normal state,
but the pain I continue to feel around me,
has my life dangling on a stake.

I feel so fragile, so frail at this time,
my energy just drains out of me,
I try to plug up these feelings that escape,
as they are not what I want me to be.

My feelings are locked in my mind,
with this pain that causes me to think,
of all the negative things to come,
and how my life is on the brink,
but I try to continue to remember my life,
with all its wonders that once was there,
and find the feelings that make me move,
and climb that ladder out there.

I have to move on, in a forward state,
with feelings of hope in my heart,
and keep to my goals,
to become once again whole,
giving my life a new fresh new start.

Personal Emotions

"WHERE'S MY PROGRESS?"

Today the pain, the movement I have, is the same as yesterday's feel,
is this the best that it will be, and how I will be real?
I exercise, and keep my mind, in a positive attitude,
but where's my progress that I need right now,
those promises it was understood.

I feel so tired, maybe a little depressed, at the rate my progress is going,
I need to begin to see some results, that reflect a positive showing.
If this is all I can improve my strength,
then tell me what to expect, I need to understand what will be,
with my body for this event.

Can I continue to cure my health, if my body just remains like this,
or is there something more I can do, to get a better control of my wits.
I have a time table that needs to be met,
or some needed relief will be gone,
so please let me know what to do to improve,
and begin to be able to move on.

If the pain that I feel, is a sign that I'll heal,
then I will continue to work very hard,
but please let me know, so a setback won't blow,
all the results that I want, that seem so far.

I won't give up now, nor get down, on what to do,
I just need to see the progress that's real,
just please let me know, other ways I can go,
to get the needed progress that I can feel.

Personal Emotions

"EMOTIONAL ILLOGIC"

These emotions I have make no sense at all, they are crazy in their own kind of way, they seem to control, any logic I have, with my tears that seem to now get in the way.

My emotions go through very strange stages each day, when all things seem to go just so right, but the emotional logic that should be right there, is not around and far from my sight.

It could be the fear that remains in my mind, or the meds that I take every day, but these emotions that come to surface to speak, are illogical in too many ways.

When I feel the love from the friend that is close, with no doubt in mind that it's real, my emotions get all goofed up inside me, when I try to respond with a feel.

I just can not be, what I want him to feel, from the depth of my heart that's for him, and I get so depressed, that my emotions are a mess, as I can not give my feelings back to him.

His logic comes across, that there is no rush for me, to be what I was before I got sick, but my emotions get involved to a point that won't absolve, the illogic that is haunting me.

I feel so bad right now, as I get ready to make my move, to do serious harm to those crazy cells, and know that I must wait, a longer while as I take, the new action that will make take me out of hell.

I have to believe that this is a small time in our two lives, that will pass and we will once again be whole, but my emotions just won't be as logical as they should be, during this time I attempt to get well.

127

Personal Emotions

" I FEEL YOUR JOY"

To be in control of your daily routines,
to feel that a movement is going your way,
you have to bring up a joy inside you,
to create such a wonderful day.

I feel your joy, I see your eyes,
they smile with a confident win,
that you are in control of your beautiful life,
from beginning to its final end.

This joy that you have spills over to me,
and engulfs my emotions for you,
It relieves all the feelings inside that I try to hide,
so I won't place a burden on you.

Your joy has a flame that ignites the air around
and makes everyone just stop and stare,
you have a special power to control,
what's around, every minute of every year.

Thanks for the experience of feeling your joy,
it's a gift that I treasure so dear,
I just want to help keep the joy flowing out,
with me right by your side for many years.

Personal Emotions

"TOUGHNESS ATTITUDE"

I couldn't be more impressed,
with the actions that you take,
to get yourself up and reaching for your goals.
It hasn't been that long,
since the verdict came along,
that tried to put you in a different place.

You have an attitude,
with a strength that can't confuse,
it reflects a toughness that most don't have,
and you work each day
so hard, making improvements each day,
that shows you have a "Toughness Attitude!"

You hide it very well,
with your softness loving spells,
that you cast upon the world around,
but I can see right through,
that you are so strong inside too,
that forms your "Toughness Attitude."

I will never worry much,
because you are so very tough,
with a warmth that exposes your love combined,
and this will always be,
the strength I see for me,
that allows me to respect just who you are.

Personal Emotions

"CAN I HOLD ON?"

I never imagined the pain I'd have,
each day that I attempt to be healed,
but every effort to conquer and succeed,
makes me wonder if I will just fail.

Can I hold on? I beg to myself to say "Yes,"
but the pain just rips deep inside,
I try to fight off all the tears that build up,
and try to put them away nearby my side.

No matter the pain, I seem to be driven,
by a determined force inside,
that tells me to continue to work even though,
the pain won't attempt to subside.

I will hold on, I do not believe,
that this pain will be forever with me,
and I will understand, that these feelings that I have,
will grow up and be gone very shortly.

Can I hold on and work real hard,
to build strength where this pain wants to live?
Can I just visualize that the pain is a sign,
that the healing is getting so big?

I will have the strength, to continue each day,
to work very hard to improve,
I just want to not have, this pain that's inside,
seems to be there all the time in this mood.

I will hold on and try to ignore,
all the pain that it takes for me to be strong,
and continue to shed all the tears in my head,
each day as I continue to carry on.

Personal Emotions

"THE HEALING WHEEL"

With movement comes an energy force,
That creates a healing process,
our thoughts combine like a super glue,
to make each movement the powerful energy circuit.
Our thoughts and actions are like a wheel,
that needs to be round and pumped,
if not the movement that we make,
will make our journey thump.

Imagine your life with a group of spokes,
that are connected to a main core,
and each of these spokes represent different aspects,
of who and what you are.
Your thoughts control the strength in each spoke,
they try to keep your wheel so round,
so keep you mind focused on healing,
it's what will keep your wheel very round.

If part of you just feels upset or depressed,
about current events that try to control,
then understand that your wheel will not move,
as it's flat or possibly not round.
Your wheel can heal, just like it can stall,
the life you care to have,
it takes an effort from your thoughts,
to be positive when seeing the bad.

Your wheel is there to help you now,
it just needs to be pumped and cleaned,
with positive thoughts that come from your heart
to make a life just beam.
So when that day comes that your wheel seems flat,
and those spokes seem just too weak,
just make your thoughts turn into strength
and see your wheel well greased.

Personal Emotions

"TRAIN YOUR BODY"

Your body expands to the limits you choose,
each day that you live your life.
Unless you stretch yourself to its limits,
you will never be able to fight.

Your body and mind will only go the limits,
that were there with you before,
so each day you need to expand what you do,
to achieve a little bit more.

The moment you become complacent and bored,
your mind will retreat back to a time,
and you will begin to regress to a place,
that only the past will be able to find.

To train your body, your soul so to speak,
to move forward to improve everyday,
requires that you just reach for new limits,
that come across your path as you play.

Love life every moment, find new things to learn,
reach for the stars when you can,
and you will discover some wondrous limits,
that get placed tight within your hand.

Each day is a test that your mind needs to take,
to allow you to grow and advance,
but you need to know that it can only happen,
when you decide to take a chance.

To risk is to learn, to try is to grow,
all we need is the effort to do,
so just train yourself to be bold all the time,
and the results will be there for you.

Personal Emotions

"REALITY SUCKS"

*I've worked so hard to improve my health,
my efforts are praised by all,
but am I just fooling myself today,
that this improvement will not be coming along.
I push myself as much as I can, some days I feel so great,
but when I pause for just a second,
I seem to reverse my wonderful state.*

*This reality sucks, it's not what I want,
I want to improve my ways,
I have to believe that my pain will subside
and eventually move away.
I am too concerned that I will hamper my goals,
these next set of jobs that I have, but what can I do,
as this pain pushes through,
all the previous improvements I've had.*

*The reality of this, is that I have a disease,
that requires a short time in my life,
to drop what I want and put up a good front,
with an effort to save my life.
The next few months will be hard on my soul,
as some changes will affect how I feel,
but I need to believe that after all is complete,
that my healing will begin to seem real.*

*So I will let, all this pain, come and go as it will,
I will concentrate hard on my tasks,
and when everything is through,
with the things I must do,
I will begin my new life that will last.
Reality sucks, but it's all that I have,
so I will face it the way I know well,
with a smile on my face, as I win this big race,
leaving this disease all alone in its hell.*

Personal Emotions

"STEPS THAT WORK"

The pain is there, it never leaves,
but something wonderful is beginning to appear,
I sense an improvement within my body,
encouragement is in the air.

I work so hard for the results I need,
now my goals are coming into view,
I need to continue to stay to my plan,
it's the only thing I can do.

The steps that work, are to not give up,
just move in a forward direction,
and make yourself see daylight ahead,
always smiling with positive attention.

To make your goals appear for you,
requires that the right steps be made,
and that you always try your best,
the results will truly amaze.

Steps that work are forward ones,
not side or backward motions,
so keep your eyes looking straight ahead,
with positive, confident notions.

Trust your progress, see it very clear,
and watch your feet begin to tap,
a dance will start inside your body,
with bounce that shows you're on top.

141

Personal Emotions

"SMILES FOR HEALTH"

What projects from your face,
reflects how you feel,
from happiness to sadness at times,
it stems from the way you expose what's inside,
of those thoughts that are attempting to hide.

To smile takes an effort,
a lot more than a frown,
but the results are ten times worth the try.
A smile is the attitude that brings out within you,
the impression your health is still alive.

It's easier to frown, to keep locked up inside,
all the thoughts that bring fear to your mind,
but a smile builds for you,
a positive attitude,
and lets you face all your fears with a style.

So smile for your health,
it's really easy to do,
just lift up your cheeks to your eyes,
and when problems appear,
don't let your smile disappear,
it's your way to make your life survive.

Personal Emotions

"PRICELESS DATES"

No matter someone's condition or mental state,
they need to have that special date.
They need to feel as normal as once they were,
to keep up their spirits when times are blurred.

As fatigue takes over the energy leaves,
causing rest to be what they feel will relieve.
But, what is needed is a caring thought,
that lifts them up, when their mood is off.

A priceless date comes when you take,
the person you see that's down,
and take them to a place they love,
that can help them remove their frown.

This time away has no structured rule,
just the care that shows its intent,
and it should be a time for all,
with all the love well spent.

A priceless date improves a mood,
it improves a mental state,
so make your effort to be thoughtful often,
and take someone on a "Priceless Date."

Personal Emotions

_____

_____

_____

_____

_____

_____

_____

_____

_____

_____

_____

_____

_____

_____

_____

_____

_____

_____

_____

_____

_____

Personal Emotions

Personal Emotions

Part Four
THE EMOTIONAL CURE

I will not try to fool you and tell you that there is a cure for cancer or the fear and anxiety you feel each day will ever go away totally. However, I will tell you that by practicing The Mind Diet Program everyday will help you find a special inner peace that will release the pressures inside your mind.

I know how well it works, I am a good example of how writing rhythm poetry calms and relaxes a trouble and worried mind. This form of journaling works for any problematic part of our emotional turmoil. I cannot remember the old person I once was. Distant memories sometimes pop into my head when I'm experiencing a wonderful moment, letting me drift back temporarily, only to appreciate what I have today.

Am I cured of my heart disease or the angina that I get periodically? The answer is no. However, I feel that my life is more relaxed. That my thoughts are less troublesome than they were before when they boiled and made me feel ill.

Do I still write my poetry when I feel sadness, anxiety and fear? The answer is yes, but understand that most of my poetry is now coming from a happier place inside my heart and is building upon the wonderful life I see for myself, even though I still have heart disease. I have taken my new life and have become a published author, in the fictional genre. It had always been a dream of mine and now I am having the most wonderful Mind Diet experiences getting lost in a fantasy world of my own creation.

My first two novels: *The Conspiracy of The Gods* and *The Devil's Poison* are my way of showing my readers that anything is possible. My background was light years from this vocation, but it became possible through the practice of the Mind Diet Program. My wife Nancy, after thirty years, is once again pursuing her love of art and is developing a line of hand painted silk scarves, original art note cards and other creative items that warms her fancy. I only tell you this as an example that even with heart disease and cancer anything thing is possible.

The last group of poetry is more upbeat and should allow you to begin to write from a positive point of view if you haven't done so already. Don't worry if you are not there yet. Go back and work on some of the previous poems so the negative emotions can have enough time to escape. The Mind Diet Program has only one goal in mind and that is to help you learn to be truthful and honest with what is going on around you and find that silver lining (The Mind Diet Experiences) that are staring you right in the face.

"MY DESTINY"

Today I embark on the final phase,
of the cure that will save my life.
With hope and anxiety that swirls all around,
as I continue to rage my fight.

My destiny is in my hands,
my attitude is the best it can be,
so I will determine the results that I want,
to create what I feel it should be.

Impatience overwhelms, it causes me doubt,
I feel sometimes all alone,
but there's no turning back for me,
from the tedious attack that I own.

It is my destiny to stay alive,
with the health that normal people have,
and show myself that what I've got,
is not so very bad.

I can't stop my thoughts of this bad dream,
the fear keeps entering my head,
but I know that I must be so tedious,
to complete what the doctors have said.

My destiny is set, to begin my new life,
with the joy and the love I can show,
I will never show in me,
a "give up" way to be,
as I complete this last cure as I go.

Personal Emotions

"I CAN'T SEE MY RESULTS"

As I work through all this pain,
the poison enters me deep,
its job to kill all those nasty cells,
doesn't allow me time to think.
I work on faith during this time of fear,
that keeps me in my living hell.

I can't see the results of what is happening,
I just proceed hoping everything works,
each day I believe that this course that I take,
will help me toward my new birth.

I have been given a new life, the opportunity for change,
a journey to find who I am,
I just need to see some results in front of me,
that reflect I will be able to stand.

There are so many choices,
with unknowns all around,
that my choices become too unclear,
I do not know the path that will make,
my life last for many years.

I just have to believe what I hear,
from the professionals around,
that my results are proceeding quite well,
so I can enjoy the time that I have,
as I go through my living hell.

I guess I will never know what tomorrow will bring,
I never was able to before,
so I will proceed everyday through this course,
with the hope I go through the right door.

Personal Emotions

"MY FRIENDS FLOPSY, YUCKY, AND POOPED"

My mind is alert, my attitude up-beat,
but my body just can't get on board,
these feeling inside, make me feel less alive,
as I attempt to move forward with my cure.

At first I felt "Flopsy,"
kind of dragging myself around,
then "Yucky" just came by one day,
and now I feel as "Pooped" as can be,
as I attempt to get through in my own special way.

I know that these friends,
are just with me right now,
and won't stay very long through this term.
I will just let them know,
that I will avoid them as I go,
with the attitude that lets me move on.

As each day progresses,
I will feel all these moods,
I will know that my rest is ok,
and I will take pleasure in,
the quiet time I'm in,
with these friends that linger with me everyday.

My body needs rest from the actions I take,
to make my life very whole once again.
I will not let this time,
get the best of me now,
as I move forward with my cure as my friend.

Personal Emotions

"WHAT CAN I DO TO HELP?"

I see your face,
your eyes that say,
"come close to me right now!"
but I am just so scared today,
I'm sorry for my frown.

You continue to do all the things you can,
but the effort is so plain to see,
I don't know just what I should do,
my feelings say give it all to me.

I see your need to have me close,
I come with my warm loving heart,
I just don't know how close to be,
or where I should just start.

Please give me clues,
if you feel you can,
I just want to comfort you so,
I see your fear,
your pain inside,
I understand as you go.

What can I do to help you now?
I am there no matter when,
just let me know what I can do,
you still are my best friend.

Personal Emotions

"I NEED SOME LAUGHTER"

Each day begins with hope that energy,
will come back to me this day,
but all I end up feeling each moment ,
is unable to be motivated or play.

I see my scars, the burn that is there,
I feel so ugly at times,
I just need to be the same as before,
to help me beam and shine.
A laugh will do, a joke of sorts,
to make my mind just sleep,
to keep me from the haunting thoughts,
that these feelings are with me for keeps.

I need to see my radiant glow, that shine that once I knew,
but these old adjectives just remind me of,
the pain I'm going through.
To laugh takes too much energy,
I feel so tired to smile,
I just want to lie down right now and sleep for just awhile.

I feel I've become just like my cats,
I sleep and poop all day,
I just can not stretch between my legs,
to add their variety to my day.

Once I felt to stay at home was a worthy goal for me,
but being home in this tired state,
is not what I thought it would be.
I guess if I must be at home,
I should understand its rules,
that rest will get me back to health
with energy and feeling good.

Personal Emotions

"WHERE HAVE ALL THESE TEARS COME FROM?"

I feel just fine, I improve each day,
I'm just tired as it's supposed to be,
but where are these tears all coming from,
this doesn't seem like normal to me.
I want to remain with energy high,
with motivation to complete each task,
but I feel the change inside of me,
afraid these feelings will forever last.

I try to hold back all my tears,
to not pass the burden away,
but as my day comes to a close,
these tears burst out their way.
I'm told to talk, to express my fears,
to not keep the tears inside,
but I just can't release myself,
to breakdown what bears inside.

Today I will begin to express,
and let myself just share,
and keep the person close to me,
up to date and so aware.
This period of time to cure myself,
is like no other time that was,
I just need to keep the faith with me,
to record this as a "was."

So as I feel the tears build up,
with the feelings that won't let me just share,
I will begin to force myself,
to allow my friends to be aware.

Personal Emotions

"SWINGING WITH MY MOODS"

Is it PMS, or Menopause,
or just a Bitchy state,
I change just like the seconds on a clock,
these moods I grow to hate.

I feel like I am on a swing,
with moods that go back and forth,
I smile then cry, with no reason why,
there's too many things that I deplore.

It has to be the treatments I have,
from torture, to poison that glows,
it has to be the reason why,
my moods just swing as I go.

I must attempt to paint a picture,
of the mood I want for me,
and see this time as a test of life,
that builds a strength that has to be.

These months that pass will make me strong,
in so many different ways,
that I should bring my moods about,
and show my smile everyday.

This is my test to show the world,
that I am in control of my own life,
I make my moods swing around each day,
with the winning smile that will win my fight.

Personal Emotions

"I SEE A STRENGTH THAT GLOWS"

Each day that passes your strength appears,
reflecting your winning state,
I feel inside a pride build up in you,
that you are winning this difficult race.

The person I see makes me so very proud,
you teach me how to live my life.
I know that your glow shines on me each day,
as I stay right by your side.

You set an example of how to deal,
with life's worst obstacles that can be dealt,
and show all around that nothing can put you down,
your energy is well spent.

Your strength just grows each day that passes,
the improvement is in the air,
your attitude has what is needed to combat,
your fear and any despair.

So see your glow, feel your strength,
your improvement comes from this wonderful mix,
and let it shine each day for you, it is your only fix.

Personal Emotions

"FROM POTPOURRI TO POOPERY"

My days used to be filled with variety and energy,
but now I just drag around as I go.
My life seemed to have many facets,
that made me enjoy my show.
But right now I just want to rest,
And gain some energy,
And be the person that once was,
Not pooped with Potpourri.

Just a little work here and a little work there,
then a nap in the middle of my day,
my life appears to be just pooped,
as my treatments keep getting in the way.

I can do so many things,
when dragged and not allowed to rest,
but my body moves slower than a snail.
I just need to realize that in all this,
my energy is going to fail,
until my treatments are all stopped,
the Poopness just won't bail.

So being just so very pooped,
will not be too bad right now,
I'll enjoy the rest until my best,
is back within its fold.

My life once had a variety,
Of things to do all day,
The potpourri will come back to me
As the fatigue just drifts away.

Personal Emotions

"MY DAYS ARE FILLED"

My routines are different, my job has changed,
during this difficult time in my life.
My day goes by in a speedy flash,
it's over with a sigh.
I like this role, it keeps me relaxed,
no pressure to make me tense,
it is the way I need to be,
to survive this unfortunate event.

How long I will be in this brand new role,
is too soon to know at this time.
I have my life and death issues to review,
this decision is only mine.
My wakeup call came in a rush,
it has warned me about my life,
and now I must determine my course,
to succeed with my current fight.

To succeed with my cure, requires less stress
and to focus on my health right now,
and if it takes some years to do,
will be the right thing for me to allow.
So what I need is to be in touch,
with the inner voice that I have,
and take this time to review my life,
and the future that won't be bad.

My days are filled with many things,
they measure a life that's new,
I need to work each day alone,
to determine just what I need to do.
So I will not be pressured by,
outside forces that want me to return to strife,
and will be forceful with all their requests,
as I continue to work on my new life.

Personal Emotions

"SMILES THAT MOTIVATE"

Motivation is what I need each day,
that makes my life renew.
Motivation gives me energy,
that helps me muddle through.

I bring a smile to my tired face,
to lift me out of bed,
then see my reflection in the mirrors around,
convinced I am not dead.

To be alive, to see the world,
each day that I have with me,
is motivation that keeps me going,
as tired as my body can be.

I'll keep my smiles upon my face,
when fatigue builds deep inside,
and use a visual motivation,
to help me believe and not hide.

I will remain so motivated,
as my days become more severe,
my smiles are needed to keep me focused,
so my positive attitude won't disappear.

So as I keep my smiles around,
I find it brings smiles right back to me,
from the people who care and love me so,
this motivation is what I need.

Personal Emotions

"I FEEL CONFIDENT"

As I look at you when your day begins,
I see a sparkle in your eyes,
I know you're defeating the ugly cells you have,
that were creating us both to cry.

Your strength, your attitude,
it's what I see in you,
that gets you through each day so confident,
in a wonderful positive mood.
You keep so positive every moment,
you don't try to hide away,
this part of you that I love so much,
allows you to be able to play.

I worry about you and the lack of control,
I have about affecting your cure,
you seem so strong,
so independent,
I begin to feel assured.

You set an example for all of us,
when we think we can't go on,
and create an environment within our world,
that makes life a happy song.

I feel so confident as I look at you,
seeing how you are taking charge,
and know that you will win at this,
no matter where you are.

Personal Emotions

"I DON'T ONLY SEE TODAY, BUT SEE TOMORROW"

It's easy to see and feel today,
with what we can touch right now,
but seeing a tomorrow bloom inside your heart,
takes some courage that's hard to swallow.

Fear for the unknown can stop you fast,
from moving forward to your destiny,
and seeing what's inside your heart right now,
can be unnerving as it can be.

You need to take life from your finished past,
with the life you see today,
and travel out beyond your fear,
to the tomorrow that's in your way.

Don't detour around, or stop to think,
just move toward your future that's there,
and see your tomorrow as a friend for you,
and reach for its helping hand.

Don't just see today as your life that is,
see your tomorrow that grows and blooms,
and take the steps that bring you toward,
the future that is waiting for you.

Each day will end, as tomorrow begins,
with unknowns that bring fear to your soul,
but reach down deep inside the tomorrows,
and watch the great person that's waiting to grow.

Personal Emotions

"YOUR COURAGE INSPIRES"

Your smiles bring forth a special mood,
something to inspire the emotional soul.
The courage you show every moment you have,
is the goal I hope I will be able to show.

Your circumstances reflect,
a reason for you to hide,
to not drive yourself to have to succeed,
And throw away your pride.
But you have the energy to pick yourself up,
that's just how you need it to be,
and create the courage in your heart,
for everyone to see.

The pride that I feel as I watch and observe,
all the efforts you make for your life,
I know just how lucky I am as your friend,
and the joy that I feel for your life.

The treatments are over,
you've done all you can,
now your energy and outlook will prevail,
I want you to know that I'll be by your side,
with support as I hold tight your hand.

Personal Emotions

"FOREVER MY LIFE"

To fight real hard for things I want,
for the things that give me joy,
requires an inner quality that comes,
from a drive I have to deploy.

Forever my life, is something that I,
just need to say everyday,
and drive myself to accomplish my goals,
no matter the darkness that's at play.

As days move on to turn to weeks,
the weeks to months and years,
forever my life will keep me on track,
so no regrets will want to appear.

Some days will seem so dark at times,
that my energy will go down the drain,
but I'll think of "Forever My Life" right now,
it will keep me in my game.

Life has no guarantees for me,
I make it what it is,
it requires work each and everyday,
that's just how it always is.

Forever My Life, is a precious thing,
I won't take it for granted at all,
and push, I'll push myself each and every day,
and sing my love of life song.

Personal Emotions

"MASSAGE MY HEART"

Pain inside from all that's around,
is tearing my soul apart,
fear overwhelms and takes over my mind,
I wish there's a way for it to stop.

At times I'm at ease, but this time floats away,
bringing back a tightness that scares me so,
I want to control my heart and my soul,
with the feelings that make me not grow old.

Please someone, Massage my Heart,
hold it tight with a softness that heals,
take me to a wonderful place,
so my mind can ease up and be still,

Softly caress my soul with the words,
that bring ease to my mind as I think,
give me the strength to renew my life,
before it is gone in a wink.

Massage my Heart, needs to come from within,
as each breath fills my lungs as I go,
Massage my Heart is the hands that I have,
to control all my fears that I know.

A release will be there, as I massage all around,
today and tomorrow with care,
and my heart will get strong, as my mind comes along,
with my heart safely held as I stand.

A change has to be, a part of the internal remedy,
that is needed to bring forth this new me,
and each day as I go, I will need to grow,
so my heart can be for once, truly free.

Personal Emotions

"YES, WE'RE GOING TO DIE"

There's been no change, the day is predicted,
when your life will go off like a switch,
no matter the news that has filled your ears,
this day will be here and the pits.

Would you go through your life in a different way,
just because you have some awakening news,
or would you proceed to this final day,
depressed or just feeling so very amused?

There is no date that can be predicted for you,
so a plan for your death can be made,
then why attempt to get depressed with yourself,
and not get on with your life everyday.

Whether it's terminal or just a fair warning,
appreciate your life that has been,
and look for the way to improve what you are,
this change has to come from within.

Yes, We're going to Die,
it was predicted the day you were born,
a life is the measure of what you have done,
and what you'll be remembered for.

Each day that you have builds upon what you've done,
the days build to weeks, then to months,
and we have the choice to add years to our lives,
being positive of what we've become.

So from this day on, make it the last day you have,
and do all you can do to be you,
and challenge yourself to attempt another day,
this attitude will pull you through.

Personal Emotions

"LIFE IS NEVER OVER"

If today comes a new beginning is formed,
so participate as if it's your last.
Build memories and joy that will fill you up
and don't dwell on your remarkable past.

Life is never over until you're in the ground,
so don't waste your time on tears and sorrow,
measure your life with smiles that show
moving forward for many tomorrows.

It's easy to go into a place that is safe,
hiding from the world that's around,
but take this time to go out of your door
to explore a new world that can be found.

Life is never over, even if you make it so,
it's just measured by the deeds that people see,
about your life-time show.
So choose the path that's right for you,
that makes your remaining days last,
It is the only life you've got,
so go out with a big belly laugh.

Personal Emotions

Personal Emotions

Personal Emotions

YOUR NEW BEGINNINGS

You should feel a change happening to you. Maybe you have become more aware of your surroundings, or you feel you can deal with your disease in a more realistic and tranquil state. It is also possible that your relationships have improved. Communication should be easier, more open, and tremendously honest. Not a painful honest that hurts someones feelings, but a constructive truth that builds a lasting relationship with you, your significant other, friends and family members.

No matter what the change has been for you, I am sure it has been positive. You now have a wonderful tool to help you through difficulties that may try to block your path as you continue to explore your new life. Use your Mind Diet Experience journal every day. Carry it with you so you can record those Mind Diet Experiences and Mind Diet Feelings that you are now seeing for the first time.

You may ask, "Why record all the wonderful sights and sounds you see?" Because it is necessary to fortify your life with what is positive everyday in your new world. Unless you keep a record of all the enjoyable experiences in your life, it can become buried when life's challenges become overwhelming. Remember, it is easy to become down and negative; unless you look for the positive aspects of your life, you can slip back into a dark world that is hungry for an unwilling playmate.

Even if you are feeling down from your disease and all hope seems lost, write A Mind Diet Poem about those feelings. If it takes two, three, or even five poems to help get you through a negative period, do it. The only control you have over your disease is your attitude and mental state.

Look for those Mind Diet Experiences, re-read your poems, and live your life to its fullest!

Thank you for sharing yourself in the Mind Diet Program. It has been a Mind Diet for me to share my love and happiness with you.

OTHER BOOKS IN
THE MIND DIET SERIES

1. *Count Your Life With Smiles Not Tears*

2. *Beyond Valentines Day, Making Love All Year Long*

To order additional books visit our website at: aminddiet.com

www.ingramcontent.com/pod-product-compliance
Lightning Source LLC
Chambersburg PA
CBHW031509270326
41930CB00006B/317